Praise for *The Complete Handbook of Quantum Healing*

"A thoughtful, comprehensive synthesis of a multifaceted approach to healing. Consider this a practical and necessary extension of the work of Rosalyn Bruyere, Barbara Brennan, and Caroline Myss."

—Belleruth Naparstek, LISW, creator of the Health Journeys guided imagery series and author of *Invisible Heroes: Survivors of Trauma and How They Heal* and *Your Sixth Sense*

"Dr. Minich's book is one of the most important books you'll ever read. More than just a 'wellness book,' *The Complete Handbook of Quantum Healing* describes how to apply the ancient wisdom of the energy centers called Chakras to everyday life in ways that can radically improve your health immediately. From the very start, she shows you how to achieve a whole new level of transformation physically, emotionally, and spiritually. You will marvel at how the small shifts and incremental changes she offers produce authentic health and healing. Dr. Minich is simply brilliant."

—Dr. Sheila Dean, author of *Nutrition & Endurance: Where Do I Begin*

"[You will find] gems of information on every page for understanding your body and how to be an ally to its healing process."

—Steve Sisgold, author of the bestselling book *What's Your Body Telling You?*

"A much-needed guide for those wanting to take advantage of the best of what many different healing modalities have to offer. It is divided by ailments, which makes it incredibly practical and easy to use. It will save you having to read countless books since all the info is distilled and organized for you. But most of all, it will give you sound advice to take responsibility for your own health, and do it successfully. I recommend this book with enthusiasm and without reservation."

—Alejandro Junger, MD, author of the bestselling book *Clean*

W9-CDT-059

"If you want to take back the power to control your own health, then you'll want *Quantum Healing* on your nightstand. With wisdom and intelligence, Deanna Minich shines the light on how we all have the ability to use our mind and spirit to heal our bodies."

—Christine Arylo, cofounder of Inner Mean Girl Reform School

"Deanna Minich has done it again! She has managed to write yet another book that is not only an easy step-by-step guide to healing but spiritually practical, too. We all have health issues from time to time, and her approach is to look more deeply at the issue so that you go to the source rather than just treat the symptom. Deanna is a true wellspring of knowledge, and this book is truly a must have. Each of her books leaves me feeling like I have gone to a beautiful retreat to refresh my soul."

—Anni Daulter, MSW, author of *Organically Raised: Conscious Cooking for Babies & Toddlers*

"This book is a wonderful integration of Eastern and Western healing disciplines. It is beautifully organized with tables, questionnaires, and diagrams to facilitate use by healers or those who need healing."

—Scott Rigden, MD, author of *The Ultimate Metabolism Diet*

"Whether your need for healing relates to a physical condition such as cancer or an emotional one such as worrying, this handbook will give you an incredible seven-part approach to regaining the balance and health you want in your life. The explanations for everything have been made very accessible, easy to understand, and clear to implement. *The Complete Handbook of Quantum Healing* needs to be in every home and healing office for quick and easy access. It truly is an amazing body of work and we are fortunate to have it."

—Krysta Gibson, publisher, *New Spirit Journal*

The Complete Handbook of

QUANTUM HEALING

An A–Z
Self-Healing Guide
for Over 100
Common Ailments

Deanna M. Minich, Ph.D., C.N.

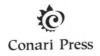

Conari Press

First published in 2011 by Conari Press
An imprint of Red Wheel/Weiser, LLC
With offices at:
500 Third Street, Suite 230
San Francisco, CA 94107

ISBN: 978-1-57324-465-7

Cover design by Maxine Ressler
Text design by Dutton and Sherman
Typeset in Warnock Pro text and ITC Bailey Sans display
Cover photograph © Le Do/iStockphoto.com

Printed in the U.S.A.

For Ian

*Opportunities to find deeper powers within ourselves
come when life seems most challenging.*

—JOSEPH CAMPBELL

Contents

Acknowledgments ix

Foreword by Cyndi Dale xi

Introduction xv

Part I
INTRODUCING QUANTUM HEALING 1

CHAPTER 1 *What Is Quantum Healing?* 3

CHAPTER 2 *The Seven Spokes of the Wheel of Quantum Healing* 11

CHAPTER 3 *The Tools of Quantum Healing* 19

Part II
YOUR A TO Z GUIDE TO HEALING COMMON AILMENTS 43

Appendices 253

APPENDIX A *Emotional Continuums* 255

APPENDIX B *Power Animals and Their Significance* 257

APPENDIX C *Flower Essences and Their Qualities* 263

APPENDIX D *Anatomical Sketch of the Human Body* 277

APPENDIX E *Positive Emotion Weekly Tracking Checklist* 279

Bibliography 281

Resources 289

Index 291

Acknowledgments

Each of us is part of the immense, intricate web of existence. We are but a mere strand, and at the same time, we are the web. When you write a book, you weave together information that becomes part of a larger pattern. During the time I spent writing this book, I have been overcome with the realization of the profundity of my past and present interactions, and within my heart, I bow in humble gratitude to those who have contributed to the greater whole of who I have become; the essence I carry has been uncovered, unleashed, and cultivated by a multitude of individuals. I could never capture everyone in a few short paragraphs, but I'll make an attempt to acknowledge the individuals who have rippled my web or helped me to be the synthesizer of intuitive and scientific knowledge.

I dedicate this book to my brother, Ian, and to him I extend a bouquet of gratitude from the inner reaches of my heart. Ian was gifted in connecting with his intuition, his soul, and his deepest side, and because of him, I learned about authenticity and exploration. Now that he is in spirit form, I feel him gently guiding and helping me find the answers I seek.

Healing is definitely in my blood, and I acknowledge and respect its origins. These origins probably go way back, but I am most familiar with the compassionate healing and grace extended through the reach of my grandmother, Elizabeth, who taught me integrity and standing one's ground. My parents, John and Sharon, have been two beautiful mentors to me and have influenced my life path greatly. I am blessed to have had their fire and air elements to bring my earthy self to life. I thank my sister, Brenda, for being the patient listener she is; she has become a force of great support for everyone in my family.

Aside from family, I thank the ripples of friends that I have met through the years—Laurie, Shonai, Ketan, Scott R., Ann, Annette, Andy, Peter, Tibor, Wieger ("Spider"), Soumya, Barbara, Brian, Nicole, Kenny, Barb S., Donna, Scott W., Epiphanio, Lyra, Kristi, Mink, Bob, Joe, Jeff B., and Jack, to name just a few. Thank you for sharing your hearts with me and letting me share my dreams with you.

I thank all the (spiritual) teachers I have met, studied with, or been influenced by: Paramahansa Yogananda, Patrice Connelly, Caroline Myss, Cyndi Dale, the teachers of the Pathways organization in Minneapolis, Louise Hay, Char Sundust, and Robin Carter. Thank you all for opening me to your techniques and wisdom, which have been woven in the collective of my spirit, heart, and body.

Thank you to the angels of the literary world—my agent, Krista Goering, who shines with brilliance and insight, and my editor, Caroline Pincus, who creates beauty and clarity within the expanse of text.

I thank my everyday, in-person teacher, Mark, for the lessons of love, balance, and support he graces me with during our time together.

And I give thanks to you, the reader, for choosing to heal, be open, and take the "high" road even when you may feel lost in the depths of confusion, pain, fear, or anger. Remember to call forth that spark within you which is good, true, and beautiful. It will light your way. Blessings!

Foreword

by Cyndi Dale

I remember the first time I was introduced to the concept of quanta. I was attending a healing workshop and practicing on another participant, analyzing each and every symptom to figure out the "one right" solution. I would will this person into wellness.

I must have looked like my youngest son does when figuring out a complex word problem, because the instructor had to stoop to peer into my eyes. "You're working pretty hard," he reflected. "I can almost see the steam coming out of your ears."

I acknowledged the observation and asked if I should be doing more.

He laughed and replied. "Why not 'go quantum' instead?"

This interaction occurred twenty-five years ago, long before words like *quantum* and *holistic* and *healing* were in vogue. Back then, vitamins practically required a physician's prescription and massage was reserved for the well-to-do in exclusive spas. Back then, to be told to "go quantum" was comparable to my kids asking me, a middle-aged woman, to break dance and merited two main reactions: "I don't get it" and "It's not happening."

We've come a long way. Medicine has expanded beyond surgery, prescription drugs, and adhesive bandages. Now vitamins are only the first step, stepchildren to vibrational medicines and herbal supplements, and massage is available at your local mall. Once considered weird, terms like *chakras, energy medicine,* and *auric fields* are almost normal table talk. But even today, many of us still wonder what it might mean to "'go quantum," especially in terms of our health.

Dr. Deanna Minich knows, and she's told us in *The Complete Handbook of Quantum Healing*. In these pages, she's bow-tied the keys to superpotent, quicksilver, quantum-sure healing, and she's done it with elegance and ease. As an energy medicine practitioner, I believe her book provides one of the most thorough and fully comprehensible approaches that I have ever seen. It is clearly aimed at *helping you feel and get better*, which is the ultimate goal of healing. Are you searching for wellness? You've merely to look up your presenting problem and follow the yellow brick road on your way to the Emerald City of quantum healing.

Of course, there is work involved. Becoming healthier takes dedication and commitment. As trite as it sounds, you can't walk without walking. Deanna, however, has discovered a way to help you secure Dorothy's magic shoes without that tedious stopover at the Wicked Witch's castle. That's what going quantum is all about—less effort, better results.

Quanta are subatomic particles, the miniscule, fast-moving energies that create and sustain physical reality. They are the building blocks of the universe, as well as your own body. If you're sick or unhappy, out-of-place quanta will leave you out of sorts. To feel better or become happier, you must shift these tiny mighty men into different positions, creating ease instead of dis-ease.

This quantum world is a strange one. If you were to spin into the quantum, you really would feel like Dorothy the farm girl dropping into the Land of Oz. Consider just three of the hundreds of quantum oddities. In the quantum world, the same particle dwells in at least two places at once—say, the future and the past (or Kansas and a dream). A particle—or an object or possibility—doesn't exist until you perceive it. And the slightest bit of effort—the right effort—can get you further than huge amounts of work.

Let's apply these three rules to healing and see what we come up with. First, quantum healing is holistic. By engaging all levels of your being, including body, mind, emotion, and spirit, you create exponential gains. It's as if you reach into the past and start erasing the problem at its origin, or stretch into tomorrow and bring your future healed state into the present. Second, by perceiving the possibilities, they start to occur. Deanna's processes help you unfold what *might* happen so it *can* happen. Third, by rearranging the foundation, the rest of the house automatically reorganizes. Fix one issue in your body, and a lot of other problems start to go away, too.

What techniques are able to accomplish these feats? For each malady, Deanna outlines several different modalities, each of which produces quantum change. She understands that a headache can stem from a tight neck, but chronic episodes could involve an array of issues, including repressed feelings, off vibrations, dysfunctional beliefs, spiritual misperceptions, poor nourishment, or (sigh) the eating of too much chocolate or some other substance. She, therefore, presents several quantum tools to help heal each condition. These tools promote mind-body interaction, but it's important to note that their intention isn't to endorse mind *over* matter, which would be a little like bullying. Rather, her techniques encourage a true partnership between the mind *and* matter.

Primary is the use of chakras as gateways. Chakras are energy bodies that link the physical with the quantum world. I've written over ten books about chakras, recording the advantage of employing them as pathways to healing. Deanna condenses everything I've ever learned and adds to it, simplifying the data so that you can easily slip into your own ruby slippers and go quantum. Once there, you invite change through processes that include visualization, affirmation, emotional realness, and the use of flower essences and power animals. The latter opens natural forces that aid the body and soul.

Healing isn't only in your mind, however. As noted, it's a partnership between your essence and your body. Employing her vast knowledge of nutrition, Deanna suggests dietary changes that nourish the body while supporting quantum mechanisms of healing. (I'm sure there are several medicinal uses for chocolate spread throughout the book.) Unique to her approach is that her dietary guidance is chakra based. This means that each recommended supplement or food item nurtures the body, but also shifts the quantum foundation, stimulating even more healing. For instance, certain liquids or nutrients will open the chakra associated with a disease, calling forth healing quanta that will get you better faster.

This book is unparalleled. It's a must for anyone interested in feeling good, but also for anyone seeking to attain optimum health. I only wish I had known how to "go quantum" years ago. I would have been able to enjoy the Emerald City a lot longer and expanded my shoe

wardrobe way beyond red slippers. May Deanna's book skip you further along the yellow brick road than you ever dreamed possible.

Introduction

When you get sick, how do you get well? What is your process for healing yourself? Is your first inclination to get a drug prescription from your medical doctor? Or perhaps you take a couple days off work to rest? Do you rush to the library for books or jump on the computer, surf the Internet, and start reading everything you can to see how you can conquer this major inconvenience? Do you join support groups and start talking to everyone you know about the condition to see what you can learn?

For the most part, I have observed that many people view healing as a nuisance, an unnecessary bump in the schedule of all the other things that need to be done. As a result, they take an approach to healing that revolves around quickly ending the physical symptom in a calculated way. In fact, like many other aspects of our lives, such as eating, driving, or working, our process for healing can often be an automatic one—one that we haven't questioned because we've grown accustomed to a certain way of going about it. We may visit a medical professional, get a prescription for a pharmaceutical drug, and hope for the best. Sometimes this approach works perfectly, while other times it may not.

The approach to healing cultivated in the twentieth century has become outdated. It has clutched to the ideas that disease meant that the body was under attack and defending the body with external substances like pharmaceutical drugs, vaccines, or other therapies was the only way of becoming well. What we didn't realize until the twenty-first century was that this paradigm isn't all that effective. Rates of chronic conditions such as cardiovascular disease, diabetes, obesity, and mental illness continued to climb despite attempts to address these conditions with the "pill for an ill" mentality. Ironically, despite technological advances in medicine, we aren't making ourselves healthier. Probably the best we are doing is extending our disabilities into a greater part of our lifespan.

Something is going on beneath the surface. Where is (are) the blind spot(s)? Where haven't we looked just yet? The real question is, *how do we truly heal?*

What science is currently telling us is that the body doesn't work in such a simplistic fashion. Terms like *network medicine* are appearing in top-tier medical journals, diseases are being connected through clusters of genes, and common mechanisms are underlying seemingly disparate diseases. The complexity of the body is emerging. Rather than being a series of linear biochemical pathways, the body is now being viewed as an interrelated web of genes, proteins, pathways, and messengers. We now know that medicine doesn't work in silos. Rather, the once-separate systems of the body envisioned by allopathic medicine are now being lumped together, as they have been in traditional medicine like Ayurveda. Instead of the nervous system, the endocrine system, and the immune system operating as distinct entities, they are being referred to collectively, in some cases, as the "neuro-endocrine-immune system."

The physical layers of medicine are coalescing into a unified whole. Along the same lines, the connection between all the layers of a human being, including both the visible and nonvisible parts of the self in the healing process—the emotions, the mind, the spiritual aspects—is being increasingly recognized. When we have dis-ease or feel imbalanced in some way physically, the entirety of who we are is affected, in addition to our physical body. Therefore, by addressing illness through one approach alone, we may miss the complexity of what is confronting us. For example, it is not uncommon to get sick right after a stressful event. If, rather than just taking an antibiotic for the resulting infection, we also examined the thoughts and emotions we had leading up to the event, we might see that there were some changes of note.

Similarly, what are our thoughts, our emotions, and state of our spirit when we are ill? Do we harbor dismal thoughts of doom and gloom, resorting to the pull of negativity, or do we hoist ourselves out of the thick of the disease enough to get perspective on what the greater lesson is? What if we saw illness as a gift, something to sink into in order to reflect on deep levels? What if we danced with our symptoms rather than feared them? How would that change our healing process?

This book came into being when I saw that people needed more than one way to heal. We are complex, multidimensional beings who require complex, multidimensional solutions. In working with others and also in my own healing process, I noticed that not everyone responds to the same modality, and some may even require myriad approaches for different conditions at select time points. Some clients would need straight nutritional advice, while others would want to see me to talk about the events going on in their lives as those events related to their physical complaint. Both groups of clients had engaged the healing process in their own unique, valid ways.

This book provides a menu of options so you can experience quantum healing on all levels for something as small as a symptom or as chronically manifest as a disease. You will be presented with a number of options, ranging from nourishment (food and dietary supplements), emotional identification and release, replacing limiting beliefs and working with power animals and flower essences, along with ideas for visualization and meditation. The reason for these particular healing modalities is that they are aligned with the various facets of the human being: the physical body, emotions, thought patterns, voice, imagination, and interconnection.

Keep in mind that this book does not present to you a comprehensive list of all the healing therapies known for the conditions indicated. I have selected the modalities based on my personal and professional experience with them and their ability to resonate with the symbolism of the energy centers (chakras). You may find that you like one therapy more than the other, which is perfectly fine. Proceed with trying it out. During your healing journey, be sure to keep a journal so you can list any subtle and profound changes that occur for you. Your sense of awareness will heighten tremendously.

Sometimes it's best to stick with just one modality and take your time with it, like the slow-moving snail, experiencing the modality to the fullest and diving deep within its confines. Other times, you may want to see what it would be like to dabble in a multitude of healing arts simultaneously (the grasshopper approach). I would encourage you to follow your intuition, or your inner voice. Listen to your body, emotions, mind, heart, and spirit as you embark upon this path. Work with a healthcare practitioner if you feel the need to have more guidance or if you want to share with another person on a confidential level.

Remember that physical changes or signs can be a ticket to go on an exquisite journey filled with learning, growth, and inner unfolding. I had a client tell me that "illness is the Western form of meditation." Therefore, it is up to you to enjoy the process of healing and to use it as a means of discovery. Wherever you are along the healing spectrum, I know that within the pages of this book lie new paths to quantum healing that can be of special benefit to you.

Note to Readers

This book is intended as an introductory, informational guide to general healing techniques and is not meant to treat, diagnose, or prescribe. The tools described herein are not for the purpose of replacing standard-of-care treatment prescribed by healthcare professionals. For any medical condition or symptom, always consult with a qualified physician or appropriate healthcare professional. Neither the author nor the publisher accepts any responsibility for your health or how you choose to use the information contained in this book.

Part I

INTRODUCING QUANTUM HEALING

CHAPTER 1

What Is Quantum Healing?

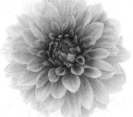

The very moment we make the choice to heal, the process is set in motion. At that point, we have many healing paths to choose from. Because of the complexity of who we are as people, sometimes it takes more than just one modality to engage the healing process. If we are trying to get to the heart of a particular issue in our lives, like combating stress or boosting our immunity, we can go at it by opening a variety of different doors—maybe by increasing physical exercise, journaling consistently, and repeating powerful affirmations daily. Or maybe just one way will work. The bottom line is that we have a multitude of options when it comes to healing, whether we're dealing with warts or arthritis, diabetes or cancer. At this point, we come to quantum healing.

Quantum is a word packed with meaning, particularly within physics: as a noun, it's the "smallest quantity of radiant energy," and as an adjective, it refers to a "sudden and significant" change. *Quantum healing is about making small changes that produce large, radiant results.* Those results may be subtle or huge, but they both give us a significant push in the direction of healing.

Quantum healing can start with something as minute as a thought, an act, a memory, an image. This seemingly small event creates a huge internal ripple effect. Take a positive thought—"I am loved." Thinking this thought can instantly change our brain chemistry. It could likely lead to changes in the flux of electrolytes (potassium, sodium) at the site of a nerve cell, stimulating the flow of serotonin (a neurotransmitter that has mood-altering effects) between nerve cells. The subsequent release of serotonin in the brain may be amplified throughout the body by triggering a network of reactions. The thought set in motion a ripple of physiological responses.

Current science tells us that the body doesn't quite work like a biochemistry flow chart, going from A to B to C in a structured, linear fashion. Rather, the human body is an organic web that interconnects

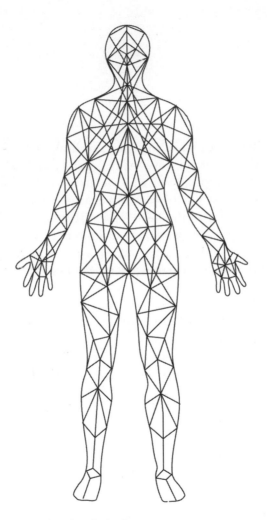

The interconnecting web within the body.

all organs and systems, so that with the flip of a serotonin switch, we see changes in other systems: heart (our heart relaxes), lungs (we breathe less shallowly), gut (we are able to digest food better), and immune system (our white blood cells respond).

When an electrical response is triggered in a part of the body, such as in the brain, the heart, or the gut, tiny cells move into action, usually starting with a change in the shape of the proteins in the cell membrane (which surrounds the cell like a wall, letting substances in and out). This change subsequently leads to proteins within the cell signaling a relay race of communication, and the message travels from protein to protein. Finally, the message makes it to the finish line, into the heart of the cell—the nucleus. The energy of this signal ultimately leads to proteins, which sit on the DNA bench, generating more proteins that will eventually be sent out of the cell and into the body at large.

Depending on the messages we feed our cells, those proteins are going to make us into glowing, radiant beings or inflamed, stressed individuals. At the end of the day, we will either have health or dis-ease, depending on the cumulative balance of the actions taken. This internal flow of events is transformative. To think that every single thing you do is shifting you at the cellular level in the direction of your wellness or disability is utterly astounding! It speaks to the profound quote by nutrition pioneer, Adelle Davis, "As I see it, every day you do one of two things: build health or produce disease in yourself."

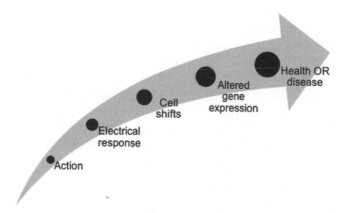

The path to manifestation of health or disease.

Of course, most of us are plenty familiar with our physical bodies, and any biochemical or physiological explanations, like the inner cascade described above, can be rather easy to digest intellectually. However, we are so much *more than our physical bodies*. We are composed of a rainbow variety of layers, some which are not even visible to the human eye. And here is another aspect of healing that involves thinking along quantum lines.

The Body-Mind-Spirit Revolution

In the past three decades or so, people have been speaking and writing about the body-mind or body-mind-spirit, implying that (1) we are more than our bodies, and (2) the body, mind, and spirit of a person are unified. There are different schools of thought on this distinction between the layers of our being, but what they all agree on is that there is more than one layer. We are multidimensional beings that have built into us varying degrees of activity. It is almost as though we are a continuum of vibration. We are woven together with different frequencies that give us our collective energy field. When we affect the *mind* (a part of us that moves quickly), we change the *emotions* (which also move quickly, but perhaps not as fluidly as mental activity; in fact, some emotions can be quite "sticky" and hang around for extended periods), and we alter the *body* (probably the slowest in its ability to change).

The systems that will be discussed in this book address the onion-like nature of our being, tapping into the body, mind, emotions, *and* spirit. Therefore, if they are practiced regularly, they are potent medicines for transforming your life and shifting your awareness.

These different ways to penetrate the heart of a disease—whether you are using colors, gems, or visualization—may not seem as foreign as they did decades ago. A survey indicates that almost 17 percent of American adults use body-mind therapies like deep breathing exercises, guided imagery, and yoga. These are most commonly used for anxiety, depression, and pain, and they are often used in conjunction with conventional medical care. Research has indicated that a majority of people (68 to 90 percent) perceive that body-mind therapies are helpful for specific conditions.

Some phenomenal results have arisen from these therapies. In a study by Annette L. Fitzpatrick and her colleagues at the University of Washington Department of Epidemiology, adults with the human

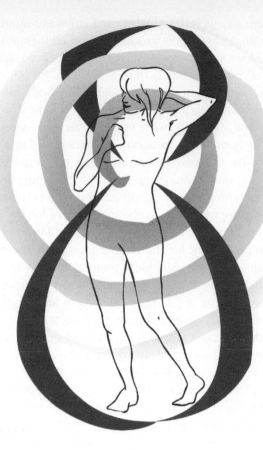

Our multi-dimensional being.

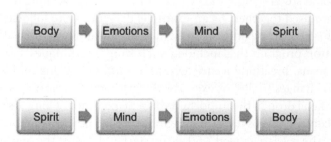

The interrelationship of body and spirit.

immunodeficiency virus (HIV-1) who used any body-mind therapy, whether psychological (support groups, individual therapy) or spiritual (prayer, meditation, affirmations, visualization), lived significantly longer (about 50 percent longer) than those who did not use these healing arts. In conjunction with prolonging life, body-mind therapies can improve the quality of life, as shown by a number of studies. People with mood disorders who followed an eight-week, audiotaped spirituality home-study program or participated in a mindfulness meditation-based stress-reduction group had improved mood (based on a mood questionnaire given at the beginning and end of study) compared with a control group given no intervention. (There was a 49 percent improvement in the mood score for the spirituality group, a 22 percent improvement for the meditation group, and a 16 percent improvement for the control group). In another study, individuals with severe psychological trauma, such as teenagers in Kosovo with high scores for post-traumatic stress disorder (PTSD), reduced their symptoms of PTSD by 20 percent after engaging in a twelve-week mind-body program encompassing techniques such as meditation, guided imagery, breathing, and self-expression through words, drawings, and movement. In contrast, the control group only experienced a 4 percent reduction in PTSD scores.

Body-mind techniques can also positively affect our physiology in measurable ways. They can lower blood pressure, reduce stress hormones, calm the immune system, and even improve blood sugar levels. Putting attention into deep breathing can cause the body to relax. Guided imagery can provide a visual template for the body to follow: if we imagine our immune system being strong, the body's defenses will respond.

Some studies show the synergy of body-mind techniques when they are used together. As an example, diabetics were followed up a month after participating in an eight-week mindfulness-based stress-reduction program that included such simple techniques as mental body scans, breathing awareness, and mindful walking and eating, but no changes to diet or exercise. Surprisingly, the participants had a beneficial drop in the important diabetic measure of long-term glucose control, glycosylated hemoglobin (also known as hemoglobin A1C). The levels averaged 7.50 at the start and 7.02 at the one-month follow-up. Participants' average arterial pressure was also reduced by six points. And if the physiological changes weren't enough, psychological measures (depression, anxiety, and general psychological distress) were also reduced by 35 to 43 percent. These results indicate how closely intertwined the body and mind are. (To see a change in the body, make a change in the mind, and vice versa!)

In another study, people with breast or prostate cancer who followed an eight-week mind-body program consisting of relaxation, meditation, and yoga reduced their levels of the stress hormone (cortisol) and reduced blood pressure, along with experiencing less inflammatory immune system activity during their continued follow-up over six and twelve months.

It is not truly understood how these mind-body therapies work so effectively. But we do know that in response to mind-body therapies like guided imagery, prayer, breathing exercises, and yoga, the body becomes open to a ripple effect of relaxation: oxygen and carbon dioxide consumption plummet, along with blood pressure, heart, and respiration rates; additionally, there are activity changes in certain areas of the brain.

Aside from these large-scale physiological changes in the body with body-mind therapies, we may also be able to impact how our genes express themselves. A fascinating study, published in 2008 by Harvard Medical School researchers, showed that 2,209 genes in people who were used to doing mind-body techniques expressed differently when compared with the same genes of people who had never practiced any of these modalities. However, when the novices were trained to do a twenty-minute mind-body technique, consisting of deep breathing, meditation, body scans, mantras, and ignoring certain thoughts, at home for eight weeks, they were able to shift 1,561 genes in a more health-promoting direction (especially with respect to how the cells deal with stress responses and inflammation).

It's rather amazing to think that we can control our genes by aligning our bodies, emotions, and minds to all work in harmony, but it's true! The more "plastic and pliable" we can remain—in our thinking, actions, body, and spirit—the more successfully we will age and achieve not only health, but optimal wellness! I have no doubt about it. Quantum healing is real. And, through this book, it's in your hands.

CHAPTER 2

The Seven Spokes of the Wheel of Quantum Healing

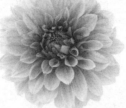

The physical parts of us are obvious because we can see them, or at least we can imagine what they look like because of anatomical sketches in textbooks. There are, however, other parts of us that are not as visible; their vibration is finer and more subtle than the dense vibration and slow frequency of the human body. We refer to this interwoven, subtle frequency as the human *energy system*. Like the circulatory system, which encompasses the action of blood running through our arteries and veins, the anatomy of the energy system is interlaced throughout the body. Ancient medical practices from India and China have depicted the energy system as a circuitry of energy threads throughout every part of the body.

In designated sections of the body, typically lined up along the spinal column and permeating through to the front of the body, there reside various energy centers. In Sanskrit, these energy centers are called *chakras* (pronounced *chuh-kras*, meaning "spinning wheels"), and they take in and distribute energy from the outside as well as harness energy from the inside and allow it to spiral outward. Although the actual physical existence of chakras has not been verified with validated technical devices, they are often perceived by those who engage in energy medicine and healing and can be useful for focusing our awareness.

The main seven chakras are correlated to parts of the physical body. However, they also have less physical and more symbolic

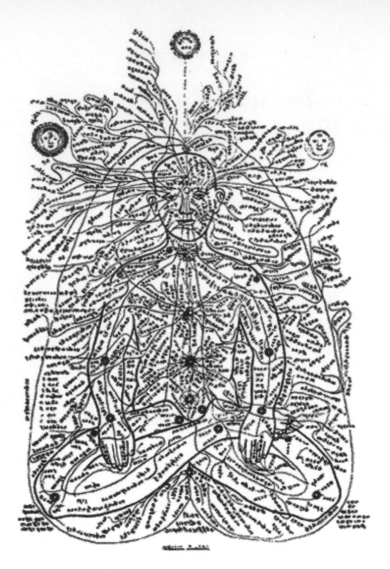

An ancient depiction of the human energy system.

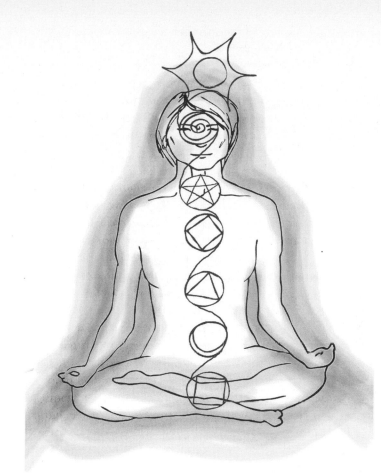

The seven major chakras (energy centers).

connections. The symbolic meanings of the chakras compose the collective of our being. If we distill down the meaning of each chakra into one word, we could make the following associations:

- Root chakra: body
- Sacral chakra: emotions
- Solar plexus chakra: mind
- Heart chakra: love
- Throat chakra: expression
- Third eye chakra: imagination
- Crown chakra: connection

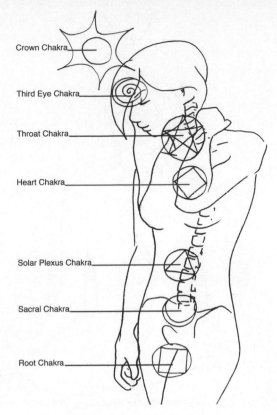

The seven aspects of our being as depicted by the chakras.

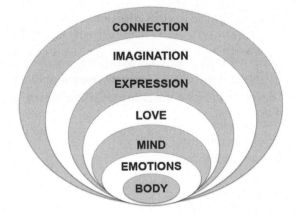

Aspects of our being to access for healing.

When we address all these parts of ourselves and not just a particular pain or symptom, we cut right through all the layers of our being and can effect a more permanent, more integrated change.

I have distilled the essential aspects of quantum healing and mapped them to these seven key areas. Here are the seven spokes of the quantum healing wheel:

1. Body/Root Chakra

General Principle: Understand the physical nature of the condition.

Specific Action: Ingest physical substances, such as foods and supplements, to correct the underlying physiological causes of the condition.

Example: Anemia is the body's inability to carry oxygen in the red blood cell due to low amounts of hemoglobin, an iron-containing protein that sits at the center of the red blood cell and latches onto oxygen. When we supplement the diet with iron-rich foods, such as spinach, or take a dietary iron supplement, we can correct for the iron level in the body so that red blood cells will be more robust and fuel the body with the oxygen it needs.

2. Emotions/Sacral Chakra

General Principle: Mine the potential emotions that are connected to a physical manifestation.

Specific Action: Substitute uplifting emotional patterns for those that are unhealthy.

Example: There is an emotional component (high fear, anxiety, worry, negative mood) to heart disease. When we combat these emotions by developing coping mechanisms or substituting acceptance for them, we may have less anxiety and less constriction, or narrowing, of blood vessels supplying the heart with blood.

3. Mind/Solar Plexus Chakra

General Principle: Uncover beliefs that underlie patterns of our behavior.

Specific Action: Substitute life- and health-promoting mental patterns for those that are outdated.

Example: If we are walking around with a belief such as "I hate myself" or "I don't accept myself" ingrained in our subconscious, we may be more apt to develop conditions that attack the self, like autoimmune conditions such as multiple sclerosis or rheumatoid arthritis. Not all autoimmune conditions are linked to these specific beliefs, but if we examine the thought on a symbolic level and how that thought might translate symbolically, this thought/belief and disease connection might be a possibility.

4. Love/Heart Chakra

General Principle: Give and receive love in a manner that enhances love of self and others.

Specific Action: Receive from nature the gift of unconditional love and healing embodied by plants (flowers).

Example: In some traditions, the planet earth is perceived as the heart of the solar system, or we are born perceived to be on this earth to learn lessons with respect to love: self love, love of another, love of people and animals, and love of nature. By using the essences of the earth, namely flower remedies/essences, we can bring ourselves back into harmony with our true nature, others, and the planet. Flower essences take raw emotions and transform them into emotional wisdom. For instance, someone who has difficulty maintaining healthy emotional boundaries may receive additional support by taking yarrow *(Achillea millefolium)* flower essence on a daily basis. This flower essence can assist in restoring a sense of self and thus reduce the need for taking on the energy of the surrounding environment, including other people.

5. Expression/Throat Chakra

General Principle: Examine verbal and written communication around us.

Specific Action: Verbalize energizing affirmations through the voice or in writing to counteract any unhealthy thoughts or emotions about the self, others, or a situation.

Example: Vocalizing and listening to the words "I trust my body's instinct," or writing these words on a sticky note and placing it somewhere you can view it every day, has a transformative effect on your subconscious mind and may help to nourish you, so that you are no longer filled with depleting, defeating thoughts about yourself.

6. Imagination/Third Eye Chakra

General Principle: Use the gift of imagination and insight to look within the body-mind-spirit landscape.

Specific Action: Visualize an intended outcome; through guided imagery, tap into the body's inherent healing properties.

Example: By repeatedly visualizing a fortified, hearty immune system that can ward off disease, and imagining we are radiating health, we may be better able to withstand a viral invasion in the future, particularly during cold and flu season.

7. Connection/Crown Chakra

General Principle: Feel connected to our inner being, to others, and to nature, in order to feel inner calm and peace and unification with all of life.

Specific Action: Meditation, prayer, silence. Connection comes in many forms; it can unfold in prayer, meditation, silence, or being in a community that is consistent with your values and beliefs.

Example: Practicing mindful eating can help you cultivate a greater connection with the origins of the food and all the hands it has passed through before it made it to the plate. When people engage in mindful eating, they are apt to develop an appreciation and awareness of all aspects of eating, and that awareness ultimately connects them to nature: the plant growing, the farmer tending to it, the elements of nature (sun, stars, moon, water) imbuing it with life, the harvester who picked it, the driver who brought it to town, the fossil fuels used in its transport, the grocer who sold it, and finally, the cook who prepared it.

Body, emotions, mind, love, expression, imagination, and connection—these parts of our being are intimately involved with our healing process. Without proper balance among these seven underlying components of our subtle and physical being, our ability to survive, emote, think, love, express, imagine, and connect become altered and out of sync. We become unwell, and we invite disease.

Through the tools provided in this book, you will open the access gates to these seven deeper parts of your nature to make way for healing. Tapping into these aspects of ourselves through the conduit of healing techniques, you will be able to access disharmony and dysfunction at deep levels of your being. Stagnant energy, ruts, and old patterns that serve you incorrectly will exit and flow out, being replaced with movement, new insights, and growth. And finally, best of all, your radiant, rainbowed, beautiful self will once again be allowed to shine through!

CHAPTER 3

The Tools of Quantum Healing

Before we move into the A to Z list of symptoms and diseases and suggestions for how to facilitate quantum healing in each, I want to introduce you to your quantum healing toolkit and how you will find these tools represented in the book. These are the approaches I find most powerful in working with each of the seven spokes of the quantum healing wheel. You see, some of the spokes are more involved with our physiological states and physical bodies, and they might respond best to foods and supplements. The spokes that operate on more subtle levels of vibration and energy tend to need emotional clearing and spiritual nourishment. As we look to invite quantum healing shifts, it is important to have tools available that are best suited to each spoke and the particular kind of healing it needs.

Tools for the Body (Root Chakra): Nourishment (Foods and Supplements)

It has been said that the physical body is the manifestation of all our thoughts, emotions, beliefs, opinions, and actions. What you see in the mirror is who you are; the physical body is the end product, so to speak. Because we can see what our body responds to, it is usually easier to start here and move backwards into the more subtle layers of our being.

There are many ways to address the physical body, and one of the most impactful ones is through the vehicle of nourishment. Not only do we make millions of choices about what and how to eat throughout our lifetimes, but we also ingest several hundred thousand pounds of food and drink. It would be unreasonable to think that our relationship to foods and eating does not impact our health! Indeed, foods and dietary supplements—such as vitamins, minerals, and herbs that we ingest over and above those from the diet—have the ability to heal our bodies. Countless studies and even medical journals are dedicated to studying the health benefits of food and food ingredients in people.

A number of population and intervention studies have observed the association between the consumption of particular foods and the occurrence of a disease. As a nutrition researcher, I spend a lot of my time reviewing the latest scientific literature and can save you the trouble of having to make your own way through them by summarizing the findings for you. Here are some overall nutrition guidelines that have repeatedly been shown to be beneficial for good health:

- An abundance of plant foods such as fruits and vegetables
- High amounts of fiber
- Low amounts of animal-based saturated fats and relatively higher amounts of unsaturated fats, like those found in olive, flax, or fish oils
- Low amounts of sodium
- Low amounts of processed foods that contain refined sugar and trans fat

You might also consider taking supplements; these should be tailored to your particular symptoms or disease. Taking supplemental vitamin D can be helpful for a number of conditions, ranging from cancer to mood imbalances. A symptom like bloating after eating might mean that your digestion could be improved with the addition of some supplemental enzymes and/or stomach acid. Your immune system function could be further enhanced in the winter months by taking a zinc supplement.

Most people think that food is needed to supply calories for the body to have energy to do something physical, and that food's physical effects stop there. The idea of food as fuel is correct—absolutely! However, when we open our eyes to the grander potential of eating—its connection to our subtle body—we optimize the what and how of our eating events. Thus, food and nutrients can have effects beyond the body. In addition to altering our body, foods impact the more subtle aspects of us—our mood and thoughts. For instance, the amount of omega-3 fats (found in fish, leafy greens, seeds, and nuts) we have in our body, particularly our brain, will determine our behavior to some extent. Low omega-3 fats in the body have been associated with an increased prevalence of depression.

The process of eating can also alter our ability to feel connected to a greater whole. If we eat in the presence of others, we may find more satisfaction from the interaction overall—from the experience of both the food and the company we are in. Or if we look at the plate before we eat and give thanks to all the aspects of nature that went into the making of the food, we may find ourselves overcome with the awe of interconnection.

Within this book, the body is addressed in two ways. First, I provide a brief description of each ailment to give you a general understanding of its manifestation on the pure physical, body level. It is also helpful to have a rudimentary understanding of your body and its basic mechanics, especially as you focus on your various organs during visualization. For this reason, a human body figure is provided in Appendix D.

Second, I provide a list of foods and dietary supplements that may be beneficial for the condition you have. These are general guidelines for the overall population and may need to be tweaked to your individual biochemistry. It would be best for you to work with a healthcare practitioner skilled in nutrition to help you adjust to doses of supplements and to create a dietary regimen just for you. If this is not possible, use the suggestions in the book as a starting point and observe how following the suggestions changes your symptoms. Keep in mind that this advice is not meant to replace that of your physician.

Tools for Emotions (Sacral Chakra): Emotion Identification

The role of emotions in symptoms and disease has been recognized for some time. For example, the number one killer of humans living in the Western world, cardiovascular disease, is typically associated with a Type A personality, or the kind of person who becomes easily stressed, angered, or provoked. People with coronary artery disease who also have a high level of anxiety have been found to be at high risk of having a heart attack or dying. Researchers have explored the triggers of cardiac events and found that negative emotional experiences or anger at work typically precede these changes in the heart.

Given how emotions directly influence our physical health, emotional release may be one way to promote better health.

Did you realize that crying is a healthy activity because of its ability to promote emotional release? An interesting study by researchers at the Nippon Medical School in Japan found that people with rheumatoid arthritis who are more apt to cry are actually in better control of their symptoms compared to those who don't tend to cry. It has also been shown that those who express their anger may experience improvements in their chronic pain. When individuals with chronic low back pain inhibited their anger, they had higher levels of muscle tension and the slowest recovery from the tension compared with those who were allowed to express their anger. It may make sense that if we harbor emotions and don't express them, they have to go somewhere. Often, they get lodged in the body, and in the above cases, the emotions seem to have become lodged in the joints or in the muscles. When emotions accumulate, we "feel" something in our body!

Expressing emotions is one way to prevent the buildup of emotions in the body. This idea was illustrated in a study with early stage breast cancer patients involving journaling practice. Those who wrote their deepest thoughts and feelings about their breast cancer, or shared positive thoughts and feelings regarding their experience with breast cancer, had decreased physical symptoms and fewer cancer-related medical appointments compared with the group of women who wrote about only facts and no feelings about having breast cancer.

As you venture down your healing path, I would encourage you to become acquainted with your emotions to the best of your ability. You may think that this is an easy task. However, when I have asked people how they feel in a particular moment, some of them are completely befuddled as to how to answer such a question. They tend to run their emotions through their intellectual filter to make sense of them. In other words, they immediately intellectualize their emotions to buffer themselves from discomforting feelings or to rationalize why those emotions are happening so that they are in control of what they feel. Others, when asked, simply shrug their shoulders that they are not sure. And still others give responses that do not address their emotional state, but some other state, like a body state

("I'm hungry," "I'm thirsty") or intellectual activity ("I'm concentrating," "I'm focused").

The more you can identify the precise emotion you are feeling, the greater your ability to work with it and to find ways to transform it, if that is your choice. The importance of being able to identify emotions was shown in a survey study on emotions and binge eating, completed by 695 college undergraduates. The results showed that having difficulty identifying and understanding emotional states, combined with limited ways to deal with emotions, was a large contributor to binge eating. If we can't make sense of our emotions and take the time to identify them, we can't come up with solutions to working with them.

The first step in chiseling away at the emotional iceberg within us is to identify the emotions that comprise it. There are several schools of thought on how emotions should be classified. The one that I find most simple and useful is one that puts them into two categories—love and fear. From these categories spring forth many different manifestations:

Love: Joy, happiness, caring, trust, compassion, truth, contentment, satisfaction

Fear: Anxiety, anger, control, sadness, depression, inadequacy, confusion, hurt, lonely, guilt, shame

People may gravitate towards the classic emotional descriptors *happy*, *sad*, *glad*, and *mad*, but these words are not rich in complexity and definition. See if you can tease out the actual underlying emotion by trying to identify more precise words to describe what you are feeling. Instead of sad, are you really disappointed, lonely, stricken with grief, or severely depressed? Instead of just saying you're mad, see if you can dialogue with this feeling of mad. Is it really anger or frustration? Is it disappointment or resentment? These emotional continuums, described both here and in Appendix A, could be therapeutic by helping you delve into, explore, and pinpoint what you are *really* feeling. When we peel away one layer of the emotion, sometimes others spring forth.

By knowing what you are feeling, you can more readily dance with it. You can express emotions in a variety of ways—by dancing, singing, making art, using your voice, crying, sharing with others,

When you feel:
SAD

Do you really feel:

isolated?
guilty?
ashamed?
tired?
lonely?
bored?
apathetic?

Defining emotional states.

and journaling, to name a few. See which way you gravitate towards. Different emotions may require a different means of expression. A client of mine likes to exercise every time she feels angry and upset and journal if she feels sad or hopeless. Another person I know likes to listen to soothing music when she feels worried.

Sometimes it's not easy to make the time to express emotions. I have many clients who complain that they do not have time in the day to feel! Or if they become emotional, they may do so in a place where it would be inappropriate to express what they feel. I say, give yourself a small sliver of time whenever you can, and if you can't conveniently express yourself, make "an emotional date" so that you will be sure to get around to expressing.

Stored, unfelt emotions are like unruly children that just want to be heard. And if they aren't heard, they start creating noise and disruption in the form of physical and emotional symptoms. If you don't believe you are feeling anything, check in with yourself to see if you have any signs of repressed emotions:

- **Fatigue.** Nothing seems to give you energy, not even sleeping or relaxing. Physical activity might give you a burst of energy, but you cannot muster the motivation to move. You start craving sugar and caffeine as an attempt to get more energy, but these substances only deplete your energy reserves further.
- **Depression.** You feel blue without knowing why, and this outlook changes your perception on life and your lifestyle. Your thoughts may become more negative and circular, and you may withdraw from your social circles.
- **Uncomfortable silence.** You feel like if you were to start talking or expressing your feelings, you might not stop crying, and you'd feel out of control. It feels safer to hold back because you're not sure what would come forth.
- **Irritability.** Becoming impatient or easily frustrated by events you may not normally react to is a signal you've got a volcano brewing inside. Because you are already full up on emotions, you can't take any more in.
- **Stomach pain.** The stomach is the hub of processing and transforming food, and its health is typically an indicator of how we are internalizing life events. When we can't digest our circumstances, or we refuse to, this energy gets stuck, causing painful ulcers and heartburn.
- **Tight throat.** If you cannot say what you mean to say, it will stay within your body. Since your throat is the vehicle of your voice, what you can't say may lodge in this area, forming a lump or uncomfortable tightness.

In the back of the book—Appendices A and E—you will find two tools to help you with emotions. See if they can help you tune into your feelings. It's almost as though we need to exercise our emotional muscles just like our physical ones. By connecting with your emotional self through written tools, you will become more used to identifying them and working with them in creative ways.

In the listings of symptoms and diseases, you will see a suggested emotion that may be associated with its underlying cause. Note that this emotion is only a suggestion. The emotion is presented as a guideline for you—a starting place or a launch pad for your feeling network. Everybody is unique. Through your own inner process, you may find that you feel emotions other than the one listed, or you may not feel any of the emotions listed, but come up with your own personalized list. This is to be expected.

Tools for the Mind (Solar Plexus Chakra): Thinking Patterns and Power Animals

Limiting Beliefs: Thinking Patterns

Our thoughts are extremely important in determining whether we are healthy or have symptoms or illness. Oftentimes, we need to step back to see what we are thinking, because we can find ourselves entangled within the "monkey mind" of all our repetitive, obsessive thoughts, many of which can be self-defeating. It is important to note the energy you put into your thinking, as each thought that has your attention will become magnified and, potentially, manifest. In a 1998 article for the journal *Archives of Dermatology,* Michael R. Bilkis and Kenneth A. Mark from the New York University Medical Center comment eloquently on this aspect of thinking:

A negative thought form can be metaphorically thought of as a "demon" who has taken up residence in a person's consciousness. It constantly makes itself known and whenever the person acknowledges it and feeds into it, the demon grows stronger. For many people, this thought eventually grows so strong that they may develop the belief that it is true and unchangeable.

If you are repeatedly thinking "I am going to lose my job," this thought may take up residence in the landscape of your mind to the degree that you may eventually begin to act out of fear and even act irrationally to the point of jeopardizing your job. Of course, this is an extreme example, but as many people have said, be careful what you wish for (or in this case, think about), because it just might come true.

Thoughts lay an energetic groundwork; when we think them, it's like adding bricks and mortar to their foundation. Eventually, the thoughts appear before us and park themselves in the field of our lives. Therefore, observe whether your thinking keeps you in the

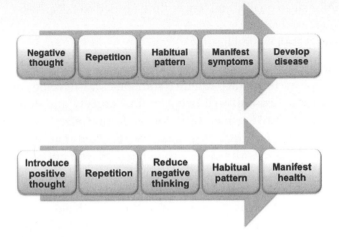

The potential of thoughts to develop into health or disease.

trenches of negativity or whether you are mired in victim thinking ("*You* are doing that to *me*"), because in the long term, such thinking may not be conducive to empowering you or promoting your health. I like to recommend policing your thoughts by spending just a couple of minutes a day not doing anything, but quickly writing down your thoughts. Note what percentages of them are life promoting and life depleting. A fun activity I recommend is the following: whenever you are having a negative thought, say aloud "cancel" or "delete" or even snap your fingers, and then rephrase the thought in a positive way. The sooner you catch yourself in that thought and correct it, the less time it has to establish a place in the home of your mind.

A number of studies have examined the role of negative thinking patterns and their effect on physical health and mood states. As you might expect, thinking pessimistically is like ingesting poison when it comes to the body. Physical health is affected in a multitude of ways by negative thought repetition (worry) and may lead to the following:

- Impaired immune system function (reduced immune-cell responsiveness under stress and trauma)
- Greater cortisol (a stress hormone) levels
- Increased heart rate and lowered heart rate variability (a risk factor for increased mortality associated with high blood pressure and cardiovascular disease)

- Poor sleep quality and longer time needed to fall asleep
- Increased fatigue
- Decreased wound healing

Habitual negative self-thinking (e.g., about body image) or rumination appears to predict whether someone will develop low self-esteem, a poor sense of well-being, and/or anxiety and depression. And negative thinking may have longer lasting effects than positive thinking. A study of college students reported that the reduced sense of well-being with negative thinking occurred not only during the thoughts, but also persisted after a several week delay, whereas positive thinking influenced the moment only and not the time that lapsed afterwards. Therefore, negative thoughts have a sticky and lasting quality to them—all the more reason to extract them from your thought database!

Some researchers have suggested that negative thinking may underlie conditions like depression and contribute to stress. In fact, mental states like depression may be masking much of the negative thinking going on underneath the mask of the mood. Also, it may be easier to resort to negative thinking if we are under stress. In one study, when individuals who had recovered from depression were asked to do a stressful cognitive task, they resorted to increased negative statements that were similar in intensity to the ones used by their tested counterparts who were still depressed. Without the added stress, the recovered individuals did not have the same degree of negative thoughts as those who were depressed. This study shows how stress can send us reeling backwards into our old thought ruts if we don't take the time to extract them from our mind.

In the book, you will find a limiting belief statement that may be connected to the thought pattern(s) underlying the symptoms or disease. These statements are guidelines only, meant to help to get you started unraveling the conscious, subconscious, and unconscious parts of you that are hooked into the body-mind-spirit issue you are dealing with.

At some point on your healing journey, I recommend doing a mind-dump exercise, where you allow yourself the physical, emotional, and mental space to let all the limiting beliefs related to a condition make their way out. Start writing these beliefs in stream-of-consciousness style, writing one limiting belief per sticky note or index card. Here are some sample limiting beliefs: "I am a failure," "No one appreciates who I am," "I am constantly confronted with challenges that prevent me from moving forward," or even "I am stuck." Enjoy the catharsis! Once you identify these limiting beliefs, survey them and see if you can distill them down to one main limiting belief. In the samples provided above, the overarching limiting belief might be "I am not worthy." From here, you can turn your limiting belief into an affirmation by positively affirming, "I am worthy" or "I am valuable." For more on affirmations, see "Tools for Expression (Throat Chakra): Affirmations" in this chapter.

Power Animals

When we are plagued with negative thoughts and limiting beliefs, we need to find ways to enhance and empower our self-esteem. One of the techniques I particularly gravitate towards because of my Shamanistic training is the use of power animals. Animal totems have special significance in the Shaman tradition, and each animal represents or embodies certain qualities. By reflecting or even meditating on these animals, we can work with them to harness our internal courage and strength. A complete list of the animals used in this text can be found in Appendix B. For each condition in the A to Z section, a power animal guide is suggested. It was selected by the traits that it imparts.

Incorporating power animals into your healing can be therapeutic, as they provide role models or even support systems, functioning much like earth-based angels.

One of my Shamanic teachers has recommended that, as we begin a quest or healing journey, we begin to notice the animals that wander, fly, or walk across our path. Simply take a second to acknowledge them and what they could be saying to you. Imagine driving your car to work one morning and seeing a squirrel running across the road in front of you. What might the squirrel mean for you symbolically? Is it time to stock up or gather your resources? What do you need to scurry from? Are you hoarding too many of your possessions, not giving enough?

The power animals that are listed for each condition are starting places for exploring working with the energy of animals. Some ways to engage with their energy might be to have a visual representation (such as magazine photo or plastic figurine) of the animal in your daily vicinity—maybe on a personal altar, on your desk at work, on your nightstand next to your bed. Read about the animals' behavior and how they live. Become knowledgeable about who they are and what they represent. You can meditate on them. You may also want to imagine they are with you in spirit form. For instance, one of the many power animals I work with is the deer, and when I feel that I am in danger, I call upon the buck to come to my rescue. I imagine the strong, tenacious qualities of a buck, especially the horns, and I immediately feel comforted.

You may also want to try dialoging with your power animal in journal form. To make their presence real, identify or create their physical characteristics and even give them a name. It's fun to even make the same noises they do!

Tools for Love (Heart Chakra): Flower Essences

Some healers contend that everything we need to heal is found either within us or within nature (plants, rocks, water, animals). Indeed, the planet is abundant with means for deep physical and spiritual healing. And whereas food and supplements primarily affect the physical being, with cascading effects on the subtle body, tools like flower essences work on the more subtle, energetic aspects of our nature. Once these layers are altered, the physical being gradually begins to change.

Thirty-eight flower essences were developed by English physician Edward Bach in the 1930s; however, other flower essences have been developed by other people since then (see Appendix C). Flower essences are liquid preparations that contain the individual energetic imprint of the flowering part of a plant (much like homeopathic remedies contain dilutions of natural or synthetic substances, like minerals or plants). The essence of the selected plant carries a vibration that corresponds at a subtle level to create a certain quality. For example, an essence of Oregon grape *(Berberis aquifolium)* helps bring forth a greater sense of trust and instinct. Because they are nontoxic and address emotional-mental aspects of our being, flower essences are safe to use, as long as we are equipped to deal with the emotional-mental changes they might bring forth.

Some published studies on flower remedies show that they may help people develop a positive outlook, but then other studies reveal no difference between those who use flower essences and those who received a placebo. These mixed results may be due to the level of subtlety flower essences work on. If an individual is looking for a dramatic change, flower essences probably aren't the best single path. However, they certainly create gentle vibratory shifts that prepare people to increase their awareness, clear their mind and surface emotions, and help with behaviors and attitudes that may impede their progress. Flower essences work wonderfully for those who tend to be sensitive to changes in their body or environment. People who have used flower essences have claimed that these essences changed their lives in quantum ways. For example:

Recently I was quite stressed out (job, terminally ill friend), and I developed problems sleeping and found focusing to be harder than normal because my mind was just too active. A mentor advised me to try the Bach Flower remedy White Chestnut. I have used these remedies for years, but never this particular one. I noticed within a day that the incessant chatter in my mind had significantly lessened. It was necessary to take it for a only few days before the negative cycle was broken.

—KAREN S.

Flower essences give me balance. I was a caregiver full time in my home for a loved one with Alzheimer's for three and a half years. She died, and I needed to find work. [I] was very stressed out and grieving. I used [the flower essences] Oak for strength, Star of Bethlehem for the loss of my favorite relative, Wild Oat to help me make the decisions I need to make at the fiftieth-year crossroad of my life, and Mimulus to help me cope with life's changes. I am doing great. Took them for six months and still use flower essences when I need balance, at least weekly. I am an unmedicated woman that relies on flower essences. I love them!

—ROBIN C.

Flower essences are excellent for work on subtle aspects of one's being—especially the emotions. Once you have identified the emotion that you need to explore, see if you can find a flower essence to match that emotion. Or, if you prefer, you can use what is presented for each condition as a starting point.

You can make your own flower essences (I will not be providing recipes here, but see the list of book resources at the back of this book for more information), or you can buy stock essences at stores or online. Options for stock essences are listed in the back of this book as recommendations. Flower essences are commonly used orally, but they can also be applied to the skin using a spray bottle, mister, or even cream, oil, or lotion. You can also add flower essences to a bath.

The classic oral dosing for flower essences is to put four drops directly under the tongue, or swirl them into water and sip the water four times per day (spread out every three to four hours). However, reduce this dose to one or two times per day for children or highly sensitive individuals. For a spray bottle or mister, four drops in eight ounces of purified water is one application. And for a cream, oil, or lotion, try seven to ten drops of flower essence per one ounce of any of these applications. If you choose to put them into a warm bath, I recommend using twenty drops of the essence.

It is important to be consistent in your usage of flower essences; periods of seven or fourteen days are optimal. To maximize their effect, combine them with other body-mind-spirit modalities such as meditation, affirmations, and visualizations. It is even better to journal about any emotional unwinding or revelations so that you can begin to process the changes that are happening to your whole being.

Tools for Expression (Throat Chakra): Affirmations

Affirmations are active, positive, declarative statements that can be used to replace negative thoughts. As you can imagine, saying aloud "I trust" instead of ruminating about how vulnerable and exposed you feel can be powerful and transforming. Repeating affirmations (several times per day for weeks or months) enables their message to occupy the conscious mind and to reprogram the subconscious mind. They are needed as substitutes for the outdated, nonserving, limiting beliefs that we have accumulated from our life experiences (starting in the uterus) or from the programming of our DNA (that is, thought patterns and mental wiring that we inherit from the family or lineage we are born into; sometimes these exist for several generations unless there is a conscious effort to remove and replace them). Just focusing on the limiting beliefs and trying to cancel them out by not thinking about them may not be as effective as actually *replacing* them. Limiting beliefs, like other thoughts, beliefs, and words, carry energy. So when we try to negate them by refraining from thinking about them, what happens is that they become like live wires, still hanging around without being dealt with. We serve ourselves best when we put that charged energy into something positive and life promoting, like an active affirmation.

Here are some testimonials from people who have found affirmations to be effective:

Positive affirmations have helped me find the space between thought and action as I healed from compulsive behaviors, like bingeing, shopping, and drinking. They are my daily medicine in curbing stress and anxiety, and as routine in my life as brushing my hair.

—LIZETTE A.

I have a client, an out of shape mother of three, who had tried every diet and exercise program possible to get in shape. I suggested trying something new. Before our workouts each morning, I would spend five minutes with her saying positive affirmations. Three months later, I talked her into doing a figure [skating] competition. She wore a gold medal in front of hundreds.

—JEFF P.

Some published research exists touting the benefits of positive statements for reducing anxiety and depression. The use of affirmations and thought-stopping techniques over a four- to six-week period was beneficial in low-income, single mothers in reducing depression, negative thinking, and stress, even after a six-month follow-up period. College students who were instructed on restructuring their negative thoughts into positive ones had better self-esteem and decreased depression.

Positive affirmations may work fairly quickly, depending on the circumstances. When study participants engaged in positive thinking before giving a speech, they had reduced anxiety about the speech and lower heart rates compared with when their thoughts were negative or neutral.

In this book, sample affirmations are provided to assist you in crafting the language you may need to unravel old patterns and reconstruct them in life-affirming ways. Feel free to create your own affirmations for any condition you are working with. The basic guidelines to designing an affirmation are to ensure that they are (1) affirming, or positive, and (2) active. Saying "I want more love in my life" may lock you into a state of wanting love rather than receiving it. Replace that sentence with this affirmation: "I receive love." Another example of strengthening an affirmation is to substitute "I deserve money" with "My life is abundant." Fewer, more potent words are not only easy to remember but also more powerful in their effect on your being.

Rooting out limiting beliefs goes hand-in-hand with using affirmations. If you are still fully programmed into a limiting belief, such as "I am unworthy," "I lack a powerful voice," or "I despise those who have more than me," it will continue to have power over you, no matter how many times you utter a positive affirmation. If you can identify the limiting belief that underlies the health condition, you can fully weed it from your mind before replacing it with a positive affirmation. Once you have identified the limiting belief and become set on removing it, positive affirmations can help to make that shift.

Sometimes as you begin reciting affirmations, there can be a hint of doubt or disbelief in the way you are saying them. This is completely normal. To be effective, affirmations have to burrow their way from your physical being into your emotional self and finally plant themselves in the garden of your mind. Repetition is the key for anchoring this new belief into your subconscious and, ultimately, into your conscious mind.

As you consistently practice using affirmations, you will find that you might go through various phases: You may begin by simply reciting the affirmation with no feeling or belief behind it. This is the physical stage, where the body utters the words, but there is no involvement from the other layers of the self. In the second stage, you could progress to saying the affirmation with a limited degree of belief and a small amount of feeling. This is the stage of warming up the emotions to the affirmation. This stage could last for an extended period of time—from days to months—depending on how much your emotions resist or accept this new paradigm.

There are varying degrees to which the affirmations will catch hold on the emotional level. Imagine a graded scale going from a deep color of disbelief to a bright color of full emotional acceptance. Once you reach the point of full emotional acceptance, you'll consistently repeat the affirmations with some oomph, and with that emotional power behind them, you'll begin to believe them.

These phases are not set in stone; rather, they provide a foundation to which you can add. For instance, you may start out with a simple affirmation such as "I accept myself," and with time, it may evolve to "I accept my ability to be authentic and creative." The key with affirmations in any stage of development is to say them like you believe them, because when you do, you will be setting in your emotional and mental bodies a new template for this new affirmation, and, one day, a change in your actions and course of life.

Here are some tips for introducing affirmations into your everyday routine:

- Write your affirmation on sticky notes or labels and put them on common objects (such as the steering wheel of your car, the telephone, the refrigerator, and the bathroom mirror.)
- In everyday exchanges with others, use key words that resonate with your end goal, so that you always keep the goal at the top of your mind.
- Act as if you have already achieved your goal by using active language.

Tools for Imagination (Third Eye Chakra): Visualizations

Based on what I have observed with others and myself, one of the most powerful ways to create what we want or need is to visualize it. By first imagining an outcome—an event, object, or state of mind or body—we increase our odds of successfully achieving it. When we have an end goal in mind, it becomes a guiding light or a general framework that the body, mind, and spirit can nestle into. Each time we revisit this framework in our thoughts and actions, it becomes more concrete until, finally, it becomes real. Conversely, without a visual image of the direction we want to head, our path can become aimless and misdirected. We may even end up in a situation that we had not anticipated or that is not desirable. As someone once said, "If we do not put energy into creating what we want, we spend that energy dealing with what we get."

The act of visualizing, or imagining, a particular outcome—often referred to as visualization or guided imagery—is an extraordinary healing art used by therapists, counselors, medical doctors, and healers of all kinds to assist their patients in relieving symptoms or moving one step closer to optimal wellness. Quite simply, visualization can be done by anyone at any time and in any place; therefore, its application has huge potential. Part of the beauty of this technique is that you can start using it as soon as today, on your own. It is simple and quick, has no negative effects, and can be done anywhere, at any time, for as little as a couple seconds or as long as hours. The practice does not have to be long in duration to see immediate results. In a one-time, eighteen-minute guided imagery session, 100 women in their thirty-second week of pregnancy experienced beneficial changes in heart rate and breathing. The fetuses must have felt the impact of the mothers' relaxed state, too, as there were significant reductions in fetal heart rates.

Individuals have used visualization practices to help treat or cure themselves of different conditions. Here are some anecdotes:

I had a cyst in my breast, and the doctors said they'd watch it. They also said these [cysts] don't really go away. I spent about two months doing affirmations and deep breathing and visualizing the cyst going away. When I went back to the doctor, it had disappeared. They took another mammogram, did more ultrasound[s], but they couldn't find it and couldn't figure it out.

—LINDA S.

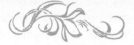

For years, I had a spot of actinic keratosis [a skin lesion] on my nose. I didn't want it frozen off because I didn't want a big red spot on my nose! I visualized it being completely healed, perfect and beautiful, during my meditation practice every day. One night, after about three weeks, I had a vivid dream that it was healed. I woke up in the morning, and the last of the little hard part [of the lesion] came off when I washed my face. [My nose] has been perfect and beautiful since!

—CINDY L.

The power of the mind to guide the body into states of wellness is not far-fetched. After all, quantum physics teaches us that matter follows thought. Scientific studies and clinical anecdotes are available to demonstrate how potent visualization exercises can be for undoing a number of ailments or health conditions; hundreds of published scientific studies validate the effects of visualization practices on everything from enhancing immune function to reducing stress, from increasing physical performance to healing disease.

Visualization is also not just about quelling symptoms; it can be integrated into one's daily life as a healthful practice. Healthy adults practicing a guided imagery and relaxation technique once a day for twenty minutes dramatically decreased their negative mood and stress and improved their positive mood and general health. These techniques were particularly effective for those who practiced them over several months.

The more you train yourself to visualize, the more readily you will be able to make the images vivid. And when they become more vivid, they are closer to manifesting. Visualization may work in a variety of ways; it might provide distraction (as in helping to relieve pain), induce relaxation, or even help the body to determine a new template for its health state. Once we have visualized a final destination, it is easier to imagine taking steps in that direction.

Additionally, practicing guided imagery can help you break habits you are ready to release. In one study, adult smokers who practiced a prescribed guided imagery exercise once daily, in conjunction with a twenty-minute, audiotaped exercise for reinforcement, over twenty-four months abstained from smoking more often than smokers who received no guided imagery (26 percent abstinence for those who used the exercises versus 12 percent abstinence for those who didn't).

Stress and Visualization

Several studies demonstrate the healing power of visualization as it connects to stressful episodes. Four weekly, forty-five–minute guided imagery sessions, done over four weeks, reduced the stress hormone cortisol in overweight Latino teens, while teens provided with no guided imagery sessions showed no changes. After twelve weeks of using guided imagery together with relaxation techniques, pregnant women experienced improved breathing and sleep, enhanced feelings of calmness, and better stress and anger management. In a study involving women undergoing radiotherapy for breast cancer, those assigned to do a relaxation and visualization therapy for twenty-four days experienced decreased stress, anxiety, and depression compared with those undergoing radiotherapy, but not using relaxation or visualization.

Pain and Visualization

Individuals with painful conditions that cannot be significantly helped by currently available medicine may be candidates for visualization therapy, especially since there are no negative side effects. People with fibromyalgia, a chronic pain condition with an unidentified cause or sustainable treatment, felt relief from their pain when they used visual imagery, combined with relaxation, for ten weeks. Another painful condition affecting more than one million Americans is interstitial cystitis (IC), which involves urinary urgency, frequency, and pelvic pain. There is little in the way of treatment for IC; however, IC patients listening to a twenty-five–minute guided imagery exercise on compact disc twice a day for eight weeks experienced reductions in pain and episodes of urinary urgency.

Visualization is for every age, and research indicates that even children can be responsive to this technique. In a two-month study with children who had recurrent abdominal pain, those taught guided imagery with muscle relaxation had a greater decrease in the number of days they had pain compared with children who practiced breathing exercises alone (82 percent versus 45 percent) after two months.

Body Function and Visualization

Visualization is not limited to reducing pain and stress. It can also help to improve the appearance and function of the body. I remember being in a seminar some years ago and listening to a doctor from China who used visualization in his practice. He talked about the powerful effects of this therapy on aspects of our physical bodies we don't think we can change. He relayed the unbelievable example of a woman who had wished to be taller. Every day, she visualized herself as taller, and after half a year, she was able to actually increase her height by almost two inches! The same doctor helped another patient to visualize becoming pregnant, as she had desperately wanted a child, and, after a year, she did become pregnant.

A collection of studies suggests guided imagery can directly impact the immune system and change the number of white blood cells, possibly by lessening stress. Women who used relaxation and guided imagery before and after surgery for breast cancer had significant improvements in their immune-cell activity compared with women who had received standard care (no guided imagery).

How to Harness the Power of Visualizations

Visualizations work much like affirmations do, although the visual stimulus makes it easier to venture into the territory of the subconscious, as such stimuli provide a map filled with lots of attractions to get to your end goal. You can practice the visualizations in this book on your own, or you can have someone read them to you. You can also record them onto tape or your computer and then play them back at your convenience.

Once you have practiced a visualization a few times, you will have it imprinted in your mind so you may not need the words anymore. You can practice guided imagery exercises anywhere. You determine if they take a couple of seconds, minutes, or hours.

The more often you do them and the longer the duration of your session, the more likely you are to see results. Some physiological variables (blood pressure, heart rate, breathing rate) can change quickly, within seconds or minutes. Other goals, like transforming the physical body characteristics and healing from a disease, may take longer to achieve. I have noticed that how long it takes to see improvements in symptoms or disease also depends on how long you have been suffering. If you tackle them right away and quickly discern their message, you can usually dissipate them quickly. If, on the other hand, you have had the symptoms or disease for twenty-five years and are just now starting to work on them with visualization practice, it may take you some months, or even years, to experience changes. However, this is not a hard and fast rule. Some people can let go of longtime symptoms or diseases quickly, especially if they are ready to embrace the change and heed the message the symptoms are communicating. The bottom line is, *the more you can get into the visualization, the more you can unravel the message of the symptoms or disease and reprogram your subconscious and unconscious mind* (which both resonate with symbology).

Tools for Connection (Crown Chakra): Meditations

Losing connection to oneself, to others, or to nature and all of life can result in feelings of loneliness and depression and even lead to symptoms and disease. Researchers have identified that a feeling of isolation, or a perception of loneliness, is associated with the risk of developing dementia. Indeed, our need for connection as humans is essential for our lives. When we feel connected and full of purpose, we are most apt to be vibrantly healthy.

A number of tools exist to give one the sense of connection with body and soul. This book will focus on meditation. Meditation is a perfect way to establish connection on many levels—body, mind, and spirit—as it allows you to filter out the background noise to make yourself open and expansive to the present moment. In fact, research suggests even a brief meditation exercise for a few minutes increases feelings of social connection and positivity towards strangers. Many people experience their aha! moments or brushes with enlightenment or the cosmos when they engage in meditation. It serves the purpose of aligning oneself and then putting oneself in perspective with all of life.

Several forms of meditation have been studied for their effects on reducing pain, stress, and anxiety and improving sleep. They may involve using a sound (such as *aum*) or mantra (healing phrase), concentration, mindfulness, focusing on an object, being in the present moment, or simply observing and releasing thoughts. Older adults with chronic back pain who participated in an eight-week mindfulness meditation study had improved sleep quality, attention, and sense of well-being, along with reduced pain. Healthy individuals who learned a meditative practice called compassion meditation, performed this practice for six weeks, and then participated in a stress test had decreased stress responses in their immune system and decreased distress scores on a mood test compared with those who didn't follow a meditation practice. In fact, the longer the time spent meditating, the better the results on mood and stress were! Researchers who compiled the results from studies on transcendental meditation (commonly referred to as TM) concluded that, on average, those who practiced TM had 4.7- and 3.2-point reductions in their systolic and diastolic blood pressures, respectively—results that are clinically meaningful.

As you will see in this book, there is flexibility in how you choose to meditate. You can decide how you'd like to weave the suggested meditative practices into your daily life. Concentration, reciting a mantra, or releasing thoughts are just a few suggested practices. Experiment with the meditations provided for the individual conditions and eventually morph them into what feels right for you. The most important aspect is to harness the meditation to feel connected, within yourself and to all of life.

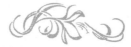

You've just been introduced to seven powerful healing tools to help you navigate your way to wellness! In the next section of the book, you will have the opportunity to try out these tools for an array of physical, emotional, and mental conditions—everything from acne to yeast infections. Of course, you can read the book from start to finish, or you might want to use it as a helpful reference, thumbing through at any time to address conditions relevant for you (or others). Let your seven-layered inner self be your guide!

Part II

YOUR A TO Z GUIDE TO GUIDE TO HEALING COMMON AILMENTS

Acne

Physical description: Acne, or skin eruptions, commonly occurs during puberty due to hormonal changes and stress; however, it may also (re)appear in middle-age adulthood, when hormones begin to shift (especially in women). When skin pores on the face, neck, back, or chest become clogged with oil, bacteria, and dead cells, an inflamed lesion results.

Energy center(s): Root, solar plexus

Nourishment: *Diet*—(1) Avoid dairy, wheat, sugar, and animal products as much as possible; (2) Emphasize low-glycemic-index raw vegetables (no white potatoes or corn), legumes, and limited fruits (no ripe bananas). *Supplements*—(1) Anti-inflammatory fatty acids such as fish oil, primrose oil, and flaxseed oil; (2) A multivitamin containing vitamins A, the B complex (especially pantothenic acid, or vitamin B5 for stress), C, D, and E, along with zinc and chromium; (3) Botanical antibacterials, like neem, and blood- and liver-support herbs, such as burdock and dandelion.

Emotion(s): Shame, anger

Limiting belief(s): I attack myself. I am at war with my identity. My life is a battleground. Change is difficult. Situations get under my skin.

Power animal: Lamb

Flower essence(s): Pretty Face

Affirmation(s): I accept who I am fully and completely. I embrace my identity. I shed what serves me incorrectly. I go with the flow of change in my life.

Visualization: Have your feet flat on the ground and take a long breath in. Imagine exhaling before you a mirror image of yourself, giving you an opportunity to examine yourself objectively. What do you see that you like about yourself? Are there physical attributes you are happy with? List those silently to yourself. Are there characteristics of your personality that are noteworthy? What aspects of your character do people compliment you on most often? Reflect on those for a moment. See yourself in communication with your environment. What appears seamless? What is challenging?

Transition your current image into one of you as a small child—innocent, curious, exploring, and quiet. This child is in perfect harmony with his/her environment, eating when needing energy, sleeping when tired, interacting with others when choosing to. Now observe your feelings about this younger image of you; did they shift from where you started? Feel tenderness and compassion for yourself in this younger form and allow those feelings to coalesce into a ball of green energy.

Use the green energy to propel the image of you as a small child into an image of yourself in the future—beyond which you are already, maybe weeks, months, or years from now. Let this image magnify all of those special features about your appearance and your character that you first recognized. Then bring in the green, compassionate energy and envelop your future self in its glow. See the green energy running through the body, from head to toes and from all fingertips. At this moment, visualize yourself in this new image as your ideal. See your absolute, perfect self in balance with all of life. Amplify in this image any personality attributes that will enable you to be successful in the world and to be comfortable in everyday living.

Once you have created and finished your new image, with your mind's eye, walk into it so it fits you perfectly, like clothing. You have been given a new skin. With your hands, feel this luxurious skin that blankets you. You notice how smooth and incredibly flawless it is. Your face, neck, and back are youthful and glowing. Give yourself thanks for this transformation. With a deep breath, affirm that you accept all aspects of your ever-changing self.

Meditation: Spend three minutes, three times a day, contemplating the aspects you like about yourself. Imagine these aspects of yourself floating through your consciousness like clouds.

Addictions

Physical description: The development of an obsession, preoccupation, or psychological dependence on a substance (e.g., drugs, alcohol, food) or activity (e.g., sex, gambling, shopping, work), which may have detrimental consequences.

Energy center(s): Root, sacral, solar plexus, heart, throat, third eye, crown

Nourishment: *Diet*—(1) Avoid addictive substances, such as alcohol, sugar, salt, fat, and caffeine, as much as possible; (2) Practice eating mindfully to control food addictions; (3) Eat high-quality protein (e.g., legumes, nuts, seeds) throughout the day to provide the body with the raw materials needed to form neurotransmitters. *Supplements*—B-complex vitamin to balance neurotransmitters in the brain.

Emotion(s): Inadequacy, isolation, insecurity

Limiting belief(s): I am unworthy. Life is beyond my control. I fear my shadow and seek to hide from my deepest thoughts and experiences.

Power animal: Lion

Flower essence(s): Gentian, Honeysuckle, Manzanita

Affirmation(s): I embrace clarity. My inner vision directs me. I am filled with light and love for myself. I am free of limitations.

Visualization: Take a full, long breath to center yourself completely. Instead of using your external vision to the outside world, open up your third eye, located in the center of your forehead between your two physical eyes. Your third eye gives you inner vision so you can see layers of yourself that are not always apparent in everyday life. At your command, your third eye becomes awake and alert, and you see before you a projection of yourself. But you see yourself differently than if you were looking into a mirror. You see your body outline, and within this outline you see a variety of colors and many cords extending out from your body. You observe any deep colors embedded within your body. You can see there are trapped emotions, thoughts, hurts within these clouded areas.

At once, you understand that these clouded colors dotting various places in your body are like magnets, and they keep you connected to the situations, events, and people who are responsible for the qualities they carry so heavily, like a burden. Having these parts lodged within you draws you to activities not conducive to the needs of your highest self, or the pure light of you that radiates as your soul. It is your choice whether or not to remove these stagnant areas feeding off your life energy.

If you choose to release them, imagine holding out a gigantic, charcoal-colored magnet in front of you. This magnet immediately attracts each of these sticky, colored clouds within you until all of them have been released from your entire being. You release the magnet into the depths of the earth, and you observe how the earth energy cleanses and transforms the energy the magnet has pulled from your being. With these blocks, hurts, and burdens removed from your inner fabric, you feel a renewed sense of energy and life.

Now your third eye shows you a movie of the possibilities and opportunities you have just opened yourself up to, and this movie looks quite different than before, when your true self was covered.

Then your third eye shifts back to your body image projected in front of you. It is clear of any darkened clouds of color, but you wonder why you have these long cords stretching out of you. They almost appear to bind you, trapping you within your life circumstances. Each cord, when you follow it out its entire stretch, is connected to a place, person, or event that continues to require much of your energy. Like the colors, these are conditions that rob you of your vital energy. However, unlike the clouds of color, these cords hook you into the continuum of your life, whether in the past, present, or future, and involve worry, fear, or anger. And they continue to drink forth your energy like straws. They want to be fed by negative energies from substances and activities. You have the choice, again, whether or not to release these life-draining cords.

You are presented with a large pair of infinitely strong steel scissors, and you are told they can cut through any material. You feel inspired to cut through the cords, one by one, with these metaphysical scissors. As you slice through them, they shrivel up and fall from your body.

You scan your projected body image one more time and find it to be clear of any obstruction, block, or any other force taking life-promoting energy from you. With a clean, deep breath of white light, you fill this body image, making it whole and pure. You can already feel a difference in your body. It feels lighter, full of joy, and resonates with your personal truth. Your third eye sinks back deep within your forehead, taking with it the projection of who you are. Your being feels free of any need to engage in any activity serving you incorrectly. You are free, you are free, like a bird flying high in the sky.

Meditation: See yourself like a bird soaring in the sky, free from any restriction, judgment, pain, or criticism. Let your breath be the air under your wings.

Adrenal Fatigue

Physical description: Adrenal fatigue is often referred to as a modern-day stress syndrome, or the inability to function optimally in everyday life due to feelings of overwhelming fatigue and an underlying feeling of being unwell. The long-term effects of cortisol (stress hormone) overstimulation and depletion are detrimental impairments in the immune system response, increased body weight, metabolic changes, and poor quality sleep.

Energy center(s): Root, solar plexus, third eye

Nourishment: *Diet*—(1) Avoid refined sugar, processed foods, alcohol, caffeine, and fatty meats, as they stress the adrenal glands; (2) Emphasize quality vegetable protein, whole grains, fish, leafy greens, and vegetables. *Supplements*—(1) Vitamin C and B complex for adrenal function; (2) Adrenal-supporting botanicals such as astragalus, Siberian ginseng, Rhodiola rosea, licorice root, ashwagandha, and cordyceps.

Emotion(s): Fear

Limiting belief(s): I am not good enough. Life fatigues me. I am constantly fighting to stay alive. I am trying to keep my life afloat.

Power animal: Porcupine

Flower essence(s): Cherry Plum

Affirmation(s): I have everything I need to succeed and live life fully. Living is effortless. I am full of all the energy I need for all I need to do, think, and feel. I am valuable.

Visualization: Feel the pulsing of urgency in your body. Note the accelerated rhythm your body beats to at this time and the current running through your nervous system, keeping you consistently wired to the point of exhaustion. Your body has been taken over by emergencies, and now it has to move faster than it can keep up with. Let's restore your body's natural rhythm, release the internal alarm, and nourish the inner self with warmth and self-acceptance.

Take a deep, full breath into the bottom of your belly. As you breathe in, notice you are also taking in calmness. The calmness you breathe in leaves no room for the weariness you feel. And with each breath to follow, you are able to exhale more and more of the fatigue you have stored up throughout your life. Your body becomes more centered, and all the acceleration you felt before has now come down several notches. You sit within your natural rhythm. Your breath keeps your nervous system and heart vibrating at a speed that feels comfortable.

At your next breath, imagine, at the same time, a laserlike beam of yellow energy filling your solar plexus region, brightening it with the brilliance of your own internal knowing. This laser light fills your empty reserves, like fuel fills a car's gas tank. It fills you completely from top to bottom until you are glowing with this pure radiance of the sun. Every cell in your body has been washed over with the luminescence of this powerful energy. You radiate this energy from every pore of your skin until all the beams you generate form a sphere around you.

This sphere buffers you from all the outer workings of society, all the emergencies that magnetize themselves to you, and all the people who demand your attention. This strong yellow orb gives you strength and confidence to move in the direction you choose. Once you are within this protective sphere, you are gifted with knowing how to use your internal resources in a way that nourishes you. The yellow light shining from within casts out from your being all outdated beliefs and opinions about how you should be and act in order to be successful and happy. Your self is now clean of anything that limits you from feeling optimal and content.

As you breathe in, your heart swells with appreciation for your newfound balance and for the release of the overdrive state you have been in for a long time. See warm, bright red clouds of energy penetrating your midback area, at the level of your kidneys. On top of your kidneys rest your adrenal glands. See the small triangular adrenals being infused with this nourishing red energy, drinking it in as though they have been thirsty for a long time. This energy has the vibration of a warrior spirit and gives the adrenals the energy they need for any emergencies that may occur. Notice the bright red color your adrenal glands have become. See them glowing with the energy of Mars, with the energy of a warrior, fighting spirit. They can be called into action as you need them, but they ask that you be selective of your calling. Their reserves are finite. Honor and protect their gift of protection and their ability to keep you safe.

Take your awareness out from your adrenals and focus it back to the rhythm of your breath. Notice the smooth flow of life-force energy that permeates you, and notice your subtle response to it and ability to take in only what you need. You are balanced and whole once again, able to deal, in a way that is seamless and effective, with all that life presents you.

Meditation: Keep a journal of what stresses you. After a week, notice if there is one thing that stresses you more than others. Meditate in search of a solution to dissolving this stressor and setting yourself free. Slowly implement the solution and continue to journal about your progress.

Aging

Physical description: In the natural course of living, the body becomes less efficient and agile in its functioning.

Energy center(s): Root, crown

Nourishment: *Diet*—(1) Reduce consumption of cooked foods (especially overcooked, fried, browned foods); (2) Emphasize smaller portion sizes (about 15 percent less than normal); (3) Focus on eating primarily nonanimal products and copious amounts of vegetables, fruits, and legumes (e.g., soybeans). *Supplements*—Multivitamin that contains folic acid, niacin, and vitamin B12 to prevent telomere shortening (an indicator of aging).

Emotion(s): Helplessness, despair, isolation

Limiting belief(s): I am old. I am worthless. I am no good for anything. I am alone and disconnected.

Power animal: Elephant

Flower essence(s): Rabbitbrush, Sweet Chestnut

Affirmation(s): I am overflowing with a love of being me. I have purpose. My connection to life is electric and feeds me with endless vitality. My body and spirit are filled with youthful vigor and a zest for life.

Visualization: You are standing in the center of a pool of gently swirling water; this water has been generated from a spring from beneath the earth and contains the primordial essence of life. The aquamarine-tinted water is clear, pure, and full of glistening life and energy. Each water droplet sparkles with the exuberance of youth and eternal vitality.

You wade in this refreshing water, splashing it on your skin, and while doing so, you notice your skin absorbs the water immediately. Your skin drinks in the youthful energy locked into the water droplets. Observe how your skin transforms within seconds by taking on a glowing appearance, free of any blemishes and wrinkles. You are like a prism radiating many beautiful, vibrant colors. You feel and stretch into this beautiful skin, gliding and dancing freely in the crystal clear water. You gently splash your eyes with the water and instantly you can see perfectly and distinctly.

Now you lie down in the water, allowing it to cover your entire body surface. With each breath you take, you can see the energy of the water permeating your body, and before long, the water in your body is replaced with the healing water of the pool. Every cell in your body is bathed in the fluid of this pure, blue, shining water.

And you are at peace. There is a feeling of contentment pervading your entire being. The water carries out all the accumulated toxins from the cells, relieving them of the burdens of aging. Their load is lightened as they are cleaned from the debris of aging, and any blocks to wellness are removed instantaneously. The tiny machinery inside your cells starts to run more efficiently, and now they glide seamlessly through their usual motions.

You are full of childlike energy. All opportunities are possible. You notice your joints feel fluid, your mind is clear of distraction and outdated thoughts. Your heart and blood vessels are clear from obstruction, and they pump through you a warm river of pure blood. Your body is once again full of renewed life and vitality. All signs of aging have been swept from your face. You are once again young in body and spirit.

Meditation: Meditate on a radiant, golden core of energy inside your low belly. For the first couple of minutes of meditation, see the sphere of energy expanding and becoming brighter with each breath, filling you with vital life-force energy. For the remaining minutes, allow yourself to bask in the glow of your life force and in the light of fulfillment.

Alcoholism

Physical description: Chronic consumption of alcoholic beverages, resulting in negative consequences, such as physiological and/or psychological addiction to the alcohol, disruptive changes in behavior (e.g., withdrawal, isolation), and poor health.

Energy center(s): Root, solar plexus, third eye, crown

Nourishment: *Diet*—(1) Remove alcohol from the diet with proper therapy, as alcohol contains a substantial amount of calories and little nutrient quality; (2) Replenish the diet with low-glycemic-index, fresh foods such as vegetables (no white potatoes), whole grains (no white rice), and moderate amounts of fruits to help bring blood sugar back into balance. *Supplements*—(1) Quality multivitamin; (2) B-complex vitamin; (3) Omega-3 fatty acids, such as fish or flaxseed oil; (4) Liver support herbs such as milk thistle (silymarin).

Emotion(s): Hopelessness, isolation

Limiting belief(s): I need to drown my sorrows. I am alone. Life is too painful for me to participate in as my true self. I give up.

Power animal: Salmon

Flower essence(s): Scotch Broom

Affirmation(s): I am enough. I trust in my Higher Will. I shed layers of my being that are incongruent with my life path. I am fed by hope.

Visualization: Close your eyes and take a few resting breaths, sinking into the moment of this time and space. With the closing of your outer eyes, let your inner vision open to a new realm. This new vision, which you always have access to, is there for you to use whenever you see fit, and you can access it at any time just by invoking it.

Imagine in front of you an exact image of yourself as you know yourself to be. Your physical body is a mirror image of the real one, and how you feel and think are replicated within your physical body. Observe yourself as you have not before, as though you are detached from the image. Notice the outer layer of this image—your physical body. And let this layer speak to you in terms of its fears around survival—around earning money, providing for shelter and food, feeling safety and trust from others, and having a community in which to anchor. What fears are present? What do you hear, or what images are being shown to you?

Notice your body's response to the effects of drinking alcohol. As information comes forth, notice the physical body is unraveling, from the head all the way down to the feet, and it burrows down into the earth beneath it.

What is now before you is your emotional body. You may not have seen your emotions in the form of an image before, but all of your collective emotions have come together to form this shape. And now you can see your emotions without the interference of your physical body. Whereas your physical body is static, your emotional body is dynamic and moving. Instead of body organs, you see patches of color circulating within this shape. You feel temperature shifts. Scan your emotional body completely, without judgment or fear. What do you intuit from this part of you? What is left hanging around within your consciousness? Are there any events that are emotionally charged that you have not yet resolved? If so, take some time to dialogue with these experiences, understand their lessons, and let a whirlwind of acceptance move through you. See how your emotional body changes when you do this.

When you have completed this process, your emotional body is swept away like rushing water to reveal another layer underneath—the part of you representing thought, your mind and intellect. It is your mental body. This image of you presents itself as a web—an entangled pattern of all of your beliefs, opinions, and thoughts. Is this a highly structured web, or is it a tangled mess filled with knots and traps? Observe the web and see if there are any particular thoughts stuck in it, like a spider's prey—especially any thoughts that may not be conducive to who you are. Old, stuck ideas or thought patterns hang around, weighing you down rather than liberating you and freeing your mind. Release these stuck thoughts by letting them unravel and fall to the ground. Now comb through the web to let go of any patterns you choose, allowing them to fall away. See how the web morphs into a new pattern. Continue to modify the web until you find a beautiful pattern, one supporting you rather than weighing you down. What do your new thought patterns say to you?

At the end, let a gentle breeze carry away the tender construct of the web you have woven, leaving behind the image of nothingness. Breathe into this space of peace, gathering in as much as you are able.

When you feel ready, bring back your renewed images before you—the physical, emotional, and mental parts of your being. Synchronize them together, creating a harmonious reflection of your true self. Envision yourself walking into the true self, filling it completely and shedding any old layers as you do so. Feel these new layers as if they were new clothing. Move around in them, becoming acquainted with your healed, renewed self.

Meditation: Meditate on the layer around your true self that the mask of alcohol has created. With each breath, imagine you shed a layer of despair and doubt, until you have relieved yourself of all superfluous, heavy, inauthentic cloaking layers. See yourself bright and brilliant before a sunset, breathing in the light of the sun's rays.

Allergies

Physical description: An allergy is developed when the immune system has a distinct reaction to an environmental trigger, such as a food eaten or exposure to mold, pollen, or dust. This contact ultimately results in a variety of physical symptoms, such as itchy skin, gastrointestinal complaints, runny nose, difficulty breathing, and sneezing.

Energy center(s): Root, solar plexus, throat

Nourishment: *Diet*—(1) Identify food allergies by working with a qualified healthcare professional; (2) Limit consumption of allergenic foods (bananas, caffeine, citrus fruits, corn, eggs, dairy products, nuts, peanuts, tomatoes, wheat and other gluten-containing grains); (3) Rotate foods every three to four days to ensure sufficient variety; (4) Avoid processed foods containing food colorings and flavorings, preservatives (e.g., sulfites; butylated hydroxytoluene, or BHT; butylated hydroxyanisole, or BHA), and artificial ingredients (e.g., sweeteners like sucralose, aspartame). *Supplements*—(1) Quercetin, bromelain, and papain (between meals) to reduce allergenic response; (2) Vitamin C and bioflavonoids to stimulate immune system function; (3) Local bee-pollen granules if you have environmental allergies (unless you have an allergy to bee-related products).

Emotion(s): Defensiveness, isolation, aloneness

Limiting belief(s): I am not at harmony with my environment. The food I eat and the air I breathe make me react to them. I distrust all that isn't from me. I feel unsafe in my surroundings.

Power animal: Turtle

Flower essence(s): Corn, Dill

Affirmation(s): I am at peace with everything inside and outside of me. I welcome new ideas, thoughts, and input and process them with ease. I determine how I react to the world. The boundaries I have created are all knowing and perfect, allowing me to take in only those things that serve my greatest good.

Visualization: Center yourself using a couple of deep breaths, and every time you breathe in, see a sparkling, golden energy emanating out through your arms and fingertips and your legs and toes. Do this until there is so much healing light within you that your body can no longer contain it, and it spills into the space around you, about five feet from your body in all directions.

You are encapsulated in a soft yellow, egglike shape consisting of healing energy and serving as your shield to the outside world. Every part of you is safe and protected by this invisible substance, which is composed of fine, vibrating molecules. It is a permanent layer of you, acting as an energetic sieve by determining what needs to enter your personal space and what needs to be released from you; in physical body terms, it is an extension of your immune system. You have the ultimate control over your immune system. It responds to your command. If you will it to protect you, it is there instantaneously in full force, radiating through you and out of you. Any type of resistance to your surroundings, which may have manifested in the form of allergies to food or to the environment, has been cast out of your physical body and your energetic space. You choose to be healthy and strong. And, in so doing, you are free of any restrictions to the air you breathe, the food you eat, and to any other factors in your environment because of your strong, able immune system.

If you had specific allergies, whether to mold, pollen, dust, or foods, imagine in your mind's eye what those looked like to your immune system. See their energetic footprint. Now imagine your immune system making peace with this substance. It no longer causes you any symptoms because you have integrated fully into your environment and you accept your surroundings.

Take a deep breath in, embracing the air you breathe with the energy of your invincible immune system. You are one with all.

Meditation: Meditate within a vision of yourself encapsulated by a thin, translucent bubble. See this layer as being permeable to only that which serves you. Breathe in harmony within this bubble. Surround yourself with this calm. Make a list of those things that cause disharmony, and journal on steps you can take to creating more acceptance.

Alopecia Areata (See Hair Loss)

Anemia

Physical description: The red blood cells do not have enough hemoglobin (a protein) to carry oxygen, resulting in fatigue and an inability to concentrate. Reasons for anemia may be blood loss, blood-cell destruction, or the inability to produce enough blood cells. The most common form of anemia is associated with iron deficiency; however, anemia can also be due to low amounts of folate and vitamin B12. (It is called "pernicious anemia" if vitamin B12 is lacking.)

Energy center(s): Root, heart

Nourishment: *Diet*—Eat iron-rich and folate-containing foods: broccoli, leafy greens, legumes (black beans, peas), prunes, raisins, turnip greens, and whole grains. *Supplements*—(1) Iron (take only if you are iron deficient; confirm your iron status by having your healthcare practitioner do a blood test). Note: Iron is best to take together with vitamin C for better absorption in the gut; (2) Vitamin B12 and folic acid (take together to prevent folic acid from masking a vitamin B12 deficiency).

Emotion(s): Apathy

Limiting belief(s): I am incomplete. I lack. The river of life within me lacks movement. I cannot carry enough energy to live.

Power animal: Bull

Flower essence(s): Mountain Pride, Olive

Affirmation(s): I am vibrant and full of energy. I move with the flow of life. I embrace myself and the world I live in. I am enough.

Visualization: With your feet flat on the ground, receive your next breath with mindfulness. Anchor this breath down into the red, flowing lava flowing within the earth's crust. This lava is the blood of the earth, nourishing the planet, keeping it warm and secure, fed with all the nutrients and healing it needs. See all the properties of the lava—its warmth, energy, life, fluidity, and vitality—enter into the vehicle of your next breath. You invite this energized breath to enter your being through the bones of your feet. At once, your feet tingle, becoming warm and invigorated with this new energy.

With your next breath, see the lava energy traveling up your skeleton into your leg bones and penetrating deep within your bone marrow. Feel the earth energy feeding your bones. The river of lava held within you continues to circulate throughout your skeleton—into your hips, ribs, arms, fingers, and skull. You feel a soothing warmth blanket your body, causing you to feel safe and secure. For the first time in a long time, you are at peace with life. Within the current of lava running through you, the earth imparts to you all the healing minerals you need, in the precise amounts you need, to form healthy blood and life-force energy: iron, zinc, calcium, magnesium, phosphorus. You accept these gifts with gratitude.

Now transition your awareness to your individual blood cells and notice that they are becoming healthy and vibrant, red and glowing with the ability to hold oxygen and life-force energy. Each new, energized red blood cell pours from the bone marrow into the circulation within the blood vessels. A river of fresh, vital red blood cells courses through your blood vessels with ease and at the perfect pace for your body. You can see them picking up and releasing oxygen where they need to. When you take your next breath, you can see the connection of the oxygen particles with the tiny, powerful red blood cell carriers, delivering oxygen to all tissues requiring it.

All layers of fatigue and depletion are shed from your physical body like layers of an onion and fall to the earth to be transformed by its healing energy into vigor and vitality. Your renewed spirit sends the lava energy that has infiltrated your bones back to its depths within the earth. Your body takes on a soft, reddish, healing glow from the inside out. You feel electric and alive!

Meditation: Meditate on the energy of red and the movement of red-colored breath in and out of your body. Do this meditation until you feel energized!

Anger

Physical description: An emotional state manifesting in mild forms such as irritation or frustration and more intense forms like fury and rage. It can lead to increased heart rate and blood pressure, along with elevations in hormones like adrenaline. Like other emotions, anger can be useful, as it can prepare the body to respond to external threats (fight or flight); however, when it is uncontrolled and suppressed, it has the potential to become unhealthy and destructive to one's well-being.

Energy center(s): Root, sacral, solar plexus

Nourishment: *Diet*—(1) Reduce warming, inflammatory foods, such as animal products, saturated fats, sugars, and salt; (2) Emphasize raw, "cooling" vegetables (e.g., cucumbers), tofu, and fruits.

Emotion(s): All forms of anger: frustration, irritation, fury, rage, depression

Limiting belief(s): I am no longer in control. Anger paralyzes my actions. I am uncomfortable with being angry or showing anger. Anger is negative.

Power animal: Dove

Flower essence(s): Aloe Vera

Affirmation(s): I act. Anger helps propel me forward. I use the fire of anger to move through difficulties. I embrace my body's reactions as important signals for me to pay attention to.

Visualization: *The most appropriate posture for this visualization is to be lying down in a comfortable position, but if that is not possible, sitting is the next best option.*

As you rest with your eyelids closed, feel if there is any tension locked within your body. Visit these places within you. Travel to them with your consciousness as though you were visiting different parts on the planet. Maybe you find you are extra tight in your chest, throat, jaws, scalp, knees. Wherever that place is, put yourself there. And dialogue with the tightness about why it is there: What does it represent? Why is it unable to release? Why does it hold back?

See if you are holding within you any unexpressed anger. Where does your anger ball up and collect? Every body will be different, and it can change each time you experience anger. But for now, find where you have collected some festering anger.

Once you have found this place, move your inner vision to your liver, which rests in the right upper quadrant of your abdomen. You can place your hand here if doing so helps you to keep your focus on this spot.

Now transform your liver energy into the form of a golden chariot, in which stands a strong warrior. The chariot is equipped with two black stallions that pull it wherever you need it to go. Your liver is the sense of movement within you; it likes to catalyze you into some action.

Now direct the chariot to the space of anger within you. Stop at this place. In a couple of moments, transform the anger into some wild horses. The warrior-driver harnesses these horses and affixes them to the chariot, so that now you have incredible momentum ready to pull the chariot. The wild horses need to release their energy and become broken in, and so the warrior directs them to move ahead, moving the chariot along with them. Allow the chariot to ride away at full steam, plowing forward through the landscape of your body and then, eventually, riding into a sunset. The chariot is being pulled by the enormous energy of the anger you withheld. It feels good to let it ride out of you.

Whenever you feel the time is right, go to wherever the chariot has stopped and examine the horses. Notice how all of them have become calm and relaxed. All anger has dissipated. Pull your awareness back to your liver. Transform it from the chariot and warrior back to its original form. Examine your body once again to ensure you have released your anger. Repeat this exercise as many times as you need in order to come to a place of peace and calm.

Meditation: Spend your meditation time journaling for three to four minutes with you anger. Listen to your anger and transcribe the monologue in your journal. After completing the exercise, take a meditative walk (preferably outdoors in nature) during which you keep an empty, clear mind.

Anxiety

Physical description: Excessive worry, fear, or dread stimulated by a feeling that external circumstances cannot be controlled or avoided.

Anxiety may be brought on by a specific event and eventually dissipate, which is a natural stress response. However, when the anxiety becomes more generalized and lasts longer, it can have detrimental physiological and psychological effects.

Energy center(s): Root, solar plexus, heart, throat, third eye, crown

Nourishment: *Diet*—(1) Remove alcohol, caffeine, sugar, and hydrogenated fats from the diet; (2) Work with a qualified healthcare practitioner to identify food allergies; (3) Eat smaller, more frequent meals throughout the day to keep blood sugar stable; (4) Engage in mindful, relaxed eating (rather than eating on the go). *Supplements*—(1) An overall, high-quality multivitamin containing B complex to ensure adequate cofactors to manufacture neurotransmitters and overall healthy metabolism, vitamin C to help with stress, and minerals like calcium and magnesium for healthy cell stimulation and relaxation; (2) Antianxiety botanicals like passionflower, hops, hawthorn, and valerian.

Emotion(s): Worry, fear, dread

Limiting belief(s): I am out of control. I want to escape. I dread what is to come. I am overwhelmed by my life. My surroundings feel unsafe.

Power animal: Panther

Flower essence(s): Aspen

Affirmation(s): I am safe. I trust that whatever happens is the only thing that could have happened. I feel confident in my ability to manage my environment. I love and trust life. I accept my response to life on all levels.

Visualization: Find your breath, and observe your breathing pattern. What do you notice? Is it stable? Erratic? Peaceful? Harmonious? How does your observation parallel your true feelings in this moment? See if you can indulge in long inhales and even longer exhales. Note whether you feel differently when you modify your breath. At all times, you can change how relaxed you feel by monitoring and adjusting your breath.

Now envision your breath like the waves of the ocean. Let your breath wash over you time after time until you have reached a point of deep, inner relaxation. Slip your awareness into the body of a dolphin, riding gracefully through the clear, blue seas. Feel a sense of freedom glide over you. The ocean water caresses the sides of your body, massaging you, and helping you to feel utterly and completely safe and at home. You shed any layers that do not serve your highest potential—any layers of anxiety or preoccupation. The sea engulfs you; the water molecules embrace your being.

You swim forward with the intention of surrendering, and into the water you release the word *peace*. Upon doing so, you see that the crystalline structure of the water molecules that bathe you is transformed uniformly, almost in a falling domino fashion, into a latticelike structure of beauty and trust. The structure of these water crystals surrounds you like a net as you swim, and it is constantly forming and reforming. You are one with the water. It nourishes and protects you.

Finally, you arrive in the shallow waters encircling a small island. You morph yourself back to your human body and walk to shore. There, you observe the sand on the beach sparkling in all directions, almost blinding your vision, yet filling you with a sense of peace and trust. As you step your foot on to the sand, you notice it is made of rainbow-colored, finely ground granules—ruby, carnelian, citrine, emerald, turquoise, aquamarine, amethyst, and diamond. You are overwhelmed by the healing radiance of this island.

You feel inclined to lie down on the fine, powdered sand, and as you do so, you are filled with the loving nature of the universe. Every particle of your physical and subtle energy bodies is aligned with the love and acceptance penetrating you from the particulates of rainbow-colored sand. Spend a couple of seconds absorbing this tremendous power of the universe. Notice how your chakras begin to align and balance themselves with the color vibrations from the sand.

You feel amazingly centered, grounded, and focused, and you decide to take yourself back to the present moment. See an electric blue outline of your empowered self before you and, when you are ready, walk into that new blueprint. Fill it with all the colors you have absorbed and all the qualities they impart. And when you are ready, open your eyes and affirm, "I am a radiant being who trusts in my nature."

Meditation: Meditate to the rhythm of your heartbeat by keeping your index finger either on the artery in your neck or on your wrist. Focus on coordinating the flow of the breath and the heartbeat.

Asthma

Physical description: A condition in which the airway tubes carrying breath in and out of the lungs become inflamed and constricted, resulting in attacks of coughing, expectoration of mucus, chest tightness, wheezing, shortness of breath, and the inability to breathe.

Energy center(s): Heart, throat

Nourishment: *Diet*—(1) Work with a qualified healthcare professional to identify food allergies; (2) Eliminate foods containing excessive food additives such as pesticides, insecticides, herbicides, and fertilizers, and also preservatives (especially sulfites) and dyes. Choose organically grown foods whenever possible, to reduce toxin intake; (3) Reduce inflammation-producing animal products (e.g., meats) and choose greater amounts of anti-inflammatory, omega-3-containing foods, such as fish (e.g., salmon); flaxseed oil; green, leafy vegetables; and nuts and seeds; (4) Avoid salt. *Supplements*—(1) Omega-3 fatty acids to reduce inflammation; (2) Vitamin C and bioflavonoids to improve immune function; (3) Quercetin and bromelain to quell inflammatory symptoms; (4) Beta-carotene for exercise-induced asthma; (5) Magnesium for better airway function; (6) Botanicals such as ginkgo biloba and licorice root, which have been shown to have anti-inflammatory, anti-allergy effects.

Emotion(s): Gripping fear to the point of feeling like you can't go on.

Limiting belief(s): I am being attacked. I am unable to surrender to the unfolding of life events. Letting go is not an option. There's no way out.

Power animal: Hummingbird

Flower essence(s): Angel's Trumpet

Affirmation(s): I surrender. I open myself to the expanse of life. I take in all life has to offer me. My life is saturated with joy.

Visualization: *It would be ideal if you could have the sound of water flowing in the background while doing this visualization.*

See yourself perched high at the top of a cliff. Looking down, you see a waterfall plunging into a collection of water, a deep pond. As you watch the flow of water spilling into the pond, you gather within you a sense of peace and calm. You observe how everything in nature has its place, that one structure moves into the next. You see the perfection of this synchronicity.

Tiny droplets rise up from the falling water, and the sunlight shining through them creates a rainbow display, almost a halo surrounding the falling water. You admire the beauty of this rainbow. With your eyes, you absorb the vibratory energy of the rainbow, bringing all the colors into your body, healing your energy centers one by one. The red falls in place in your lower body, close to your tailbone, and cascades down your legs. The gentle, yet vibrant, mist of orange penetrates through you to find its home in your low belly, nourishing your creativity and emotions. The golden, shimmering yellow in the rainbow glides down to a point several inches above your navel, at the level of your stomach. It infuses you with power, self-esteem, and energy. The healing green light enters and travels almost magnetically to your heart area, filling you with a sense of love and peace. Once you connect with the green energy, you are endowed with the insight that everything in your life appears to be connected to love, leaving no room for fear. Blue-indigo droplets of mist weave their way into your neck and head, allowing you to open up to a feeling of expansiveness and insight in your thoughts and imagination.

After you have taken in the essence of this rainbow fully and completely, you become part of the water, slipping into the stream, the beautiful trickling waterfall making its way to its source. Imagine your body has transformed from its current physical form into an ocean. Let yourself go entirely into the flow of water. Give yourself the freedom of having no defined form, other than seeing yourself as a collection of tiny water droplets reflecting a deep, blue-green color.

As you inhale, your chest rising to receive breath, see yourself merging with the spring of water below. All of your being, tiny droplets, move and dance amongst all the other water molecules, and you feel a part of the whole, trusting in the movement of the water and also in its existence. Your mind is free of questions and any lingering thoughts. Your emotions are calm within you. You have become one with the universe, and you trust where you are and what you have become.

Meditation: Meditate on the rhythm of the breath moving into and out of you. Focus on the simplicity of this action; notice the process of receiving and releasing. Let it be magnified in your consciousness. Afterwards, journal on how you are receiving and releasing ideas, opinions, emotions, events, people, and objects in your life. Where is there a lack of flow?

Atherosclerosis

Physical description: A condition in which the artery walls become inflamed and hardened due to an infiltration of fat and immune cells (a substance collectively known as plaque). Continued progression of plaque buildup can lead to blockage of the artery and eventual heart attack or stroke.

Energy center(s): Heart

Nourishment: *Diet*—(1) Eat as if you live in the Mediterranean region of Europe by emphasizing fresh vegetables, particularly green, leafy vegetables; whole grains (purple/black rice is particularly beneficial); lean meats (preferably fish); olive oil; fresh herbs (e.g., rosemary, oregano); and modest amounts of fruit; (2) *Pay attention to fats:* Reduce saturated fat, typically found in animal products like meat, butter, and milk. Avoid trans fats (identified on food labels as "partially hydrogenated oils"), usually found in processed, nutrient-depleted foods like cookies, cakes, doughnuts, and crackers. Emphasize omega-3 fats like those in fish, leafy greens, nuts, and seeds. Use olive oil for cooking and flaxseed oil for salad dressings; (3) Drink black or green tea, pomegranate juice (high in antioxidants), and/or tomato juice (for lycopene). *Supplements*—(1) A high-quality multivitamin containing folic acid, niacin, and vitamins E and C; (2) Magnesium for overall heart health; (3) Botanicals such as garlic, grape-seed extract, and pine bark extract may also be helpful.

Emotion(s): Anger, callousness, feeling emotionally stiff and inflexible

Limiting belief(s): I am blocked to love and joy in my life. I am constantly challenged by my circumstances. My anger continues to fester. I am resistant to change and flow.

Power animal: Lion

Flower essence(s): Blackberry, Dandelion, Honeysuckle, Walnut

Affirmation(s): I expand to the beautiful flow of life. I embrace love. I am open to giving and receiving in equal measure. My life is full of joy. I remain flexible. Courage flows through my heart and into all of my actions.

Visualization: Imagine yourself in a sunlit valley, at the bank of a fast-moving river. The river sparkles as the sunlight plays off the surface of the water. This river appears to be full of life and vitality. It is so welcoming that you decide to embark upon its current with your durable canoe.

You ease you way into the water, feeling secure in the canoe. You paddle yourself to the middle of the river, and then you simply let the current take you. It moves at a comfortable pace, not too fast. As you flow on the river, you notice all the life teeming around you: The trees lining the riverbank are spotted with magnificent eagles. Hawks glide overhead in the cloudless sky. Silver-scaled salmon can be seen brushing past your canoe. You are filled with a sense of joy and completeness, taking in all of nature's beauty. You breathe in the natural air and the vibration of perfection. You continue to glide down the river with your hands outstretched in the canoe, taking in this marvelous event, feeling the happiness of the moment saturate your being.

A couple miles forward, you notice the river is obstructed by a cluster of fallen trees, which has collected a variety of debris. The flow of the water is slowed down in this part of the river because of the blockage. You decide to paddle off to the side of the riverbank to see if you can help. At that moment, an eagle appears to you. It tells you that the only way to help bring back the healthy flow of the river is for you to feel love in your heart for the river. You decide not to question the eagle's remark, as it is a wise, regal bird and seems to know so much about the river already. It is almost as though the eagle has been waiting for you to arrive so you can help.

You sit down on the riverbank on a patch of green grass. You are close enough to the river for you to dangle your feet in its pristine water. Your breathing allows you to feel calm and centered. The energy of the green grass beneath you comes into your low spine and travels up to your heart area. Your heart unfolds with the energy of green goodness.

And, with your heart open, you are able to enter into a feeling of love and expansiveness. You remember a time in your life when you felt loved and you gave love to others. With these memories, your heart expands manifold, and the love you feel in your heart space permeates your being. In sync with your breath, you extend your arms outward to give out this love to the river waters. As you swing your arms back to your heart, you receive the pure essence of the river, and it gives your entire energy a soft, rosy glow.

Your body is tickled by the exchange of love with the river, causing every cell in your body to giggle with delight and joy. This light energy travels down your legs and into your feet, which are immersed in the cool, soothing river. Your love trickles through your feet and fills the river, making its way over to the obstruction. The fallen trees and debris begin to spiral in your love. They begin spiraling quickly, creating a whirlpool-like movement that transforms them into more love energy. The river takes on a beautiful, iridescent, pinkish hue. It has become a magical river, flowing only with the energy of love.

You become so enamored with the river once again that you dive in, swimming with the flow of sparkling water. The eagle you previously met travels overhead and thanks you for transforming the river. You smile, and your heart fills with endless joy.

Meditation: Place both hands over your heart and, as you inhale, feel your breath expanding your heart chambers and branching blood vessels, relaxing them and making them feel soft and supple. As you exhale, release all tension held in your circulatory system into your hands as you open them up to the space in front of you. Continue with this pattern of breath until you feel relaxed and heart centered.

Atopic Dermatitis (See Eczema)

Attention-Deficit (Hyperactivity) Disorder (ADD, ADHD)

Physical description: A display of consistent inattentive, impulsive behavior, identified typically in children (but may carry on into adulthood) and may be accompanied by hyperactivity. May ultimately impact learning ability, social interactions, and, if it continues into adult life, workplace performance.

Energy center(s): Solar plexus, third eye

Nourishment: *Diet*—(1) Exclude highly processed foods containing added sugar and unhealthy additives like dyes, preservatives, and artificial sweeteners (e.g., soft drinks, high-sugar juices, snacks); (2) Work with a qualified healthcare professional to identify food allergies; (3) Increase fiber to help bind in the gut toxins taken in from the environment; (4) Include high-sulfur foods such as cruciferous vegetables, garlic, and onions to assist with the binding of heavy metals taken in from the environment. (There is a relationship between learning disorders and heavy-metal accumulation in the body.) *Supplements*—High-quality multivitamin (avoid those containing allergens, dyes, or sweeteners).

Emotion(s): Denial, doubt, isolation

Limiting belief(s): My life (or the lives of others around me) is (are) chaotic. I fear boredom and aloneness. I will be noticed if I am frenetic and busy. My thoughts overwhelm me.

Power animal: Mouse

Flower essence(s): Aspen, Dill, Fairy Lantern, Madia, Rosemary, White Chestnut

Affirmation(s): I am focused and clear. I resonate to information that serves my highest good. I am blessed with the gift of discernment.

Visualization: Explore the territory of your mind by putting your consciousness into a tiny, mobile vehicle. Drive the vehicle into your mouth, letting it sit on your tongue, and then imagine there is a portal to your mind opening at the roof of your mouth.

You enter the portal gently, and you see before you roads and highways leading in all directions. There are intersections, spiraling ramps, parking garages, and buildings. But, mainly, there are roads. And you see a number of them are crowded, and the traffic is stagnant, as if in a traffic jam. Other roads are more fluid, and cars are traveling a dangerous 100 mph or more on them, moving at such rapid speeds that they appear as blurs. There are even some roadside fires and accidents awaiting help. Pollution and smoke are rising from various places in the landscape.

You survey the scene at large, and you find yourself in the thick of much chaotic activity. Only you alone can change this scene, as this is your territory.

The first thing you decide to do is to relieve any and all traffic jams. You do this by ensuring there are enough roads and seamless connections between these roads. You are able to have this work done quickly by simply deciding to do it. The scene shifts; more roads are added, and junctions are put in place to help with transitions from one place to another. The traffic begins to flow and move at a steady, safe pace where there were traffic jams. Much congestion is removed, and you feel at greater peace.

You then observe cars traveling at dangerously high speeds and you decide to rewire their machinery from a distance, enabling them to travel at a maximum speed of 65 mph. You have the ability to change the speed at which you want these cars to travel, but for now, it feels comfortable for you to have them going slower.

Now the situation in the landscape of your mind is feeling much more under control, with less congestion, stagnation, and speed. It feels balanced. There are still some accidents, smoke, and pollution you'd like to tend to. Through the roof of your mouth, you breathe in air containing clearing and healing energy, and you send it to provide assistance to all the accidents and to blow through any smoke and pollution still hovering over the scene of your mind. With your exhale, you release any oxidative damage in your mind, any fuzziness or cloudiness about your way of thinking, and any inability to focus completely on a task.

Now you step back and observe your mind from a distance, and you notice it appears flowing, focused, unstuck, and conducive to going places. Feeling a sense of peace, you decide to go for a ride within your mind. The sun is out. No worries obstruct your movement. You move on through your mind, fascinated at all the intricacies and sights at the roadside. Let yourself travel and be in the moment.

When you are ready, let your vehicle come back to its point of entry, the portal at the roof of your mouth, and exit through your mouth. Your consciousness steps out of the car and into every cell of your being, fully and completely. Your mind is clear and focused.

Meditation: Watch your thoughts intently in meditation. Allow them to move in slow motion, and then speed them up as fast you'd like them to go. While you do this, remain detached and free from their influence. Practice this exercise on a daily basis to be able to manage your thoughts and to enhance focus and concentration.

Autoimmune Disease

Physical description: The body's immune system becomes imbalanced to the degree that it begins to attack itself. Specifically, the immune system creates antibodies to the genetic material (DNA) or to other proteins in the body. The end result is that one or more tissues (e.g., skin, joint, nerves, gut) in the body become vulnerable to this attack, and symptoms (e.g., rash, joint swelling, nerve dysfunction, gut inflammation) result.

Energy center(s): Root (Depending on the specific condition, other chakras can be involved. For instance, because it involves the nervous system, multiple sclerosis also connects to the crown chakra.)

Nourishment: *Diet*—(1) Work with a qualified healthcare professional to identify food allergies; (2) Eat more whole, raw foods (vegetables like leafy greens, nuts if you're not allergic, and fruits) in place of highly processed, high-sugar food items (e.g., snack foods, soft drinks); (3) Reduce animal products high in inflammatory fats (e.g., fatty meats, dairy products); (4) Eat more cold-water fish (e.g., salmon, mackerel). *Supplements*—(1) High-quality multivitamin; (2) For immune system support, vitamins C and D, zinc, selenium, probiotics; (3) To reduce inflammation, digestive enzymes (taken between meals), an omega-3 oil (fish or flaxseed oil) supplement, ginger, turmeric, hops extract.

Emotion(s): Anger, feeling attacked from within

Limiting belief(s): I put others before myself. I am unworthy. I am unsatisfied with who I am and how I make my way in this physical world.

Power animal: Deer

Flower essence(s): Evening Primrose, Goldenrod

Affirmation(s): I am worthy. I am attentive to my own needs. I accept all aspects of myself, including those that concern my ability to be safe and survive in this world. I love and accept myself.

Visualization: Go within and find your breath. Find the rhythm of your breath and sit on it like a magic carpet to take a ride into who you are. Every cell in your body needs the oxygen you take in, so with your conscious awareness focused on your breath, you will travel into the terrain of your cells.

Pick an area of your body you'd like to explore, and once you are there, make yourself very small so you can be on the same level as a cell. The cell is guarded by a slippery wall that lets things in and out. Observe whether your cell wall has integrity: Does it have boundaries? Or is it too rigid or too permeable, letting everything that comes its way enter?

Slip into a cell and notice all the players within the cell: the protein-manufacturing machinery, the powerhouse of the cell that makes energy for the cell to live, and lots of little cell messengers relaying signals on the outside in. Each part is doing its function.

Note whether your cells are too busy or too slow and delayed, and if so, with your intention, ask that the cell be properly tasked. Once you do this for one cell, the change shuffles into place for all cells.

Now, as you move deeper within the cell, you come across a fence, and on the other side of the fence is the cell treasure—your spiraled DNA! You open the gate to enter the realm of your DNA—the pure essence of *you*. And you might notice it may not be properly positioned. Maybe it is too tightly coiled together or too loose. Maybe you see some proteins clinging to it that shouldn't be there. Some parts of your DNA seem as though they have been under attack—quite possibly by your own immune system.

At this time, dialogue with your DNA to discover what it needs to be restored to health. Do the proteins your body makes need to be altered or modified? Does your immune system need to be less aggressive? Does your DNA feel protected within the cell? Respond to whatever answers you receive from the origins of you. What does your body need at a cellular level? What will change the functioning in your entire body? Acknowledge the answers you receive with openness. Honor and thank your DNA. Envision it wrapped in a halo of white, protective light to prevent it from being damaged. As you do this, all DNA in your body takes on the same glow of white light. Any damage to the DNA is shed like old skin and transforms into protective proteins, which act as guards around the DNA structure.

Your immune system is rewired so it is now protective and defensive on your behalf, rather than attacking you unnecessarily. See all parts of your anatomy becoming strengthened—your immune system, digestive system, nervous system, respiratory system, reproductive system, musculoskeletal system, integumentary (skin) system. You begin to feel more vibrant, whole, and supported by your body structure. All parts are working in harmony with the others.

Meditation: Meditate using the mantra "I love and accept myself." Journal about ways you can be more loving to yourself, and implement at least one of these ways.

Back Pain

Physical description: Acute or chronic pain in the lower back, middle back, or upper back that may be due to a variety of causes: nerve and muscle dysfunction, degenerating vertebral discs, poor posture, improper lifting, and/or arthritis, to name a few.

Energy center(s): Root, sacral, solar plexus, heart, throat

Nourishment: *Diet*—Reduce animal products high in inflammatory fats (e.g., fatty meats, dairy products) and eat foods rich in anti-inflammatory fats (e.g., salmon, mackerel, walnuts, flaxseed meal, leafy greens. *Supplements*—(1) Omega-3 fats (fish or flaxseed oil) for chronic pain; (2) High-quality multivitamin containing vitamin C, bioflavonoids, and B complex; (3) Digestive enzymes taken between meals to reduce inflammation; (4) Anti-inflammatory botanicals such as devil's claw, willow bark, ginger, turmeric.

Emotion(s): Feeling overwhelmed and/or unsupported, untrusting

Limiting belief(s): I am unsupported. I am carrying burdens and worries about survival all by myself. The weight of the world is upon me. Life is back breaking.

Power animal: Turtle

Flower essence(s): Baby Blue Eyes, Elm, Oak, Quince

Affirmation(s): I move through life with ease. I am supported financially, emotionally, and spiritually. I release all burden.

Visualization: *When you do this visualization, make sure your back is comfortable.*
Close your eyes and imagine yourself lying face down on a massage table. Surrender and sink into the table as much as you can. Give thanks to yourself for taking the time to indulge in the healing of your back.

Take a deep breath, noticing how your breath arches your spine like a wave in the ocean. With each breath up to the fourth breath, you feel the energy of four healers surrounding you—one at your head, one at either side, and one at your feet. They are silent, but you can feel the phenomenal magnitude of their presence.

The healer on your left side represents the air element, including new beginnings, illumination, youth, and freedom. With her breath, she blows into your back the gift of newfound resiliency. She lays a feather on your back as a symbol of your ability to take flight whenever you feel the need. She imparts the wisdom that you are liberated by the choices you make.

The healer at the base of your feet, who represents the fire element, puts his hands on the soles of your feet, and you feel warmth rising in your legs and quickly making its way to your spine. This tingling, fiery feeling of healing wraps around your spinal column like a pole and radiates out into adjoining muscles, loosening them up. The warmth melts any tension harbored in your muscles. Your back begins to feel significant relief.

To your right is the healer holding the essence of the water element. He lays a warm sheet of water on your back and under the front of your body. Your back is the middle layer of this warm watery sandwich, which moves you gently back and forth, creating some vibration that loosens up the extracellular matrix. The healer then commands the water to gather together in a conical form and funnel through the top of your head and down the stretch of your back; tiny rivulets cascade out from the main funnel running through your spine. The cool water relieves your back of any inflammation.

And finally, at your head, stands the stoic healer responsible for the earth element. She holds within her hands a basket filled with stones, precious gems, and sand. Very thoughtfully, she places them with loving intention on your back. Two warm, medium-sized stones the size of the palm of your hand are positioned on either side of the base of the spine in order to serve as reservoirs of any painful memories or events that have lodged here and led you to have difficulty with money, survival, security, and trust. One long quartz wand is fitted along the length of your spine to absorb any negativity. Four small, shiny marcasite spheres are positioned on either side of your spine all the way up to your shoulders to absorb any feeling of having to "watch your back" and taking in the hurts inflicted by your interactions with others. And finally, two malachite stones are put on your shoulders, releasing you from the tension of burden.

Each healer puts out a hand towards your body, and, with the aid of air coming as a white light through the healer on your left, the flame of fire comes as a red energy through the hand of the healer at your feet, the wave of water swims as blue energy through the hand of the healer on your right, and the enlightenment of the earth pours as green energy through the hand of the healer at your head. All energies come together and weave into a long stretch of supportive energy, like a blanket for your back, to be there for you at all times. Your back feels renewed by the four elemental healers, and you give them each a unique expression of gratitude.

When you are ready, rise from the table, and mentally affirm, "I am supported."

Meditation: Put your concentration at the base of your spine, at your tailbone, and breathe in a cooling, healing breath, directing it to this part of your back and allowing your back to release and be invigorated. Exhale any tension, burden, or residue that feels painful. Work your way up your spine, slowly ending in the upper neck (cervical) area. This breath-spine meditation can take as little as a couple of minutes for maintenance care or, optimally, as long as thirty to sixty minutes if you need to focus on active pain release.

Baldness (See Hair Loss)

Benign Prostatic Hyperplasia (See Prostate Problems)

Bladder Infection (See Urinary Tract Infection)

Blindness (See Vision Loss)

Bloating (Abdominal)

Physical description: Abdomen feels distended and tight, causing discomfort. Potentially due to any number of reasons: low stomach acid and subsequent protein indigestion; low pancreatic enzymes, resulting in reduced breakdown of carbohydrate, protein, and fat; constipation; excessive gas; overeating; bacterial overgrowth; in serious cases, tumors.

Energy center(s): Sacral, solar plexus

Nourishment: *Diet (if bloating is due to food issues)*—(1) Eat small portions of food at each sitting to allow for proper digestion; (2) When you eat, eat to the level of being 70 to 80 percent full; (3) Eat simple meals—especially monomeals, in which you have just one food at a time; (4) Eat slowly and mindfully, spending at least twenty minutes on larger meals; (5) Avoid raw nuts and seeds, as they can be difficult to digest and many people have allergies to them; (6) Work with a qualified healthcare professional to identify food allergies. *Supplements*—(1) Betaine hydrochloric acid (acid to break down protein in the stomach; use under the supervision of a healthcare professional); (2) Try digestive enzymes with a meal to enhance the breakdown of nutrients. Also take them between meals to assist with any inflammatory processes in the gut; (3) Probiotics to reestablish healthy gut flora.

Emotion(s): Worry, feeling overwhelmed, unable to "digest" life events emotionally

Limiting belief(s): I have difficulty processing my life events. I lack the ability to transform my life into meaning and action. There are some things I cannot digest or accept. I resist.

Power animal: Cow

Flower essence(s): Dill, Filaree, Indian Pink

Affirmation(s): I digest life with ease. I am easygoing. I take in only that which serves my highest self. I digest life experiences in a way that is whole and complete for me.

Visualization: Close your eyes and put your hands on the bloated region of your abdomen. Sit with your abdomen for a couple of seconds, monitoring the movement of breath in and out of that region.

Envision that in your abdomen you have a large, buoyant balloon. It sits inside, causing discomfort. Imagine you have a magical pin, which doesn't hurt you, but is able to perforate the balloon just enough to slowly let out all the excess air. You puncture the balloon carefully, and as you do, you realize your abdomen is slowly releasing all the excess air. Ensure that your exhales are deep so you can release what is no longer needed. With your hands, feel your abdomen deflating slowly.

Now imagine you ingest some natural plant enzymes to chew up the remnants of the balloon. The balloon becomes smaller and smaller until it finally disintegrates, and as it does, you begin to feel more room in your abdomen. The plant enzymes work on anything else in your gut that remains undigested. See your gut processing any residual foodstuff or any emotional event that was hard to digest.

Give yourself a couple of seconds for the gut to clear, and after it has done so, clean your gut with a dose of white and pink liquid light that you drink in. This healing liquid light travels through your stomach, balancing your stomach-acid production, and zips through your small intestine, stimulating sufficient production of enzymes from the pancreas and proper flow of bile. It then travels into the lower gut and wipes out any excessive bacteria, bringing your colon's microflora back into balance. Finally, the liquid light exits through the rectum, swirling its way through and out.

Move your hands on your abdomen in a clockwise motion, gently massaging it, and affirm to your belly, "I digest life experiences in a whole and complete way for me."

Meditation: Put your awareness at the level of where you feel bloated. With each breath you take, see this area begin to radiate out golden rays of light. In your mind's eye, notice the particulates of light, or photons, extending out from this center, and representing the stuck, undigested energy within. Now choose whether you keep these photons within or you disperse them to outside your belly. Breathe the light back into a concentrated core in your gut. Keep your breath focused here for the remainder of the meditation.

Blood Pressure, High (Hypertension)

Physical description: Increased resistance in the arteries when blood is pumped through them by the heart. Typically assessed by measuring the peak pressure when the heart contracts (systolic blood pressure) and relaxes (diastolic blood pressure). According to the American Heart Association, high blood pressure (also called hypertension) is defined as a systolic pressure of greater than or equal to 140 millimeters of mercury (mm Hg) and a diastolic pressure of greater than or equal to 90 mm Hg. High blood pressure increases the risk of cardiovascular disease and stroke.

Energy center(s): Root, heart

Nourishment: *Diet*—(1) Eat more plant foods relative to animal foods. (Relative to nonvegetarians, vegetarians consume greater amounts of nutrients like fiber, vitamins, and minerals, which are essential for blood pressure regulation, and lesser amounts of saturated fat, which has been linked to heart disease and stroke.) (2) Emphasize leafy green vegetables, which are high in minerals, to balance blood pressure; (3) Avoid processed foods containing sugar and trans fat, as these foods predispose one to increased blood fats and the risk for obesity and type 2 diabetes. (4) Reduce salt intake. *Supplements*—(1) High-quality multivitamin containing vitamins C and E and the B complex, as well as important minerals like calcium and magnesium; (2) Coenzyme Q10; (3) Garlic.

Emotion(s): Frustration, anger, feeling overwhelmed

Limiting belief(s): I am under immense pressure. I am constrained and unable to be free of my situation. Do it perfect or not at all. It's my way or the highway!

Power animal: Eagle

Flower essence(s): Aloe Vera, Cherry Plum, Dogwood, Willow

Affirmation(s): I let go of the outcome. I embrace the flow of life. I move effortlessly in all I do. I am flexible.

Visualization: Take a deep breath to prepare you for this visualization to address high blood pressure in your body. And, if needed, take another lung-filling breath.

When the time is right, go within and observe how your body responds to the word *pressure.* What types of images, words, sensations, or feelings do you get in your body upon hearing or visualizing that word?

Now scan your body to find where there are places of pressure living within you. Where are there clusters of unmet expectations, open-ended goals, letdowns, and sheer disappointment? Where is there the stress of having to make a living and surviving in the physical world amidst an obstacle course of deadlines, time constraints, parental obligations, spouse commitments?

Use your inner eye to sift through your body compartments to locate where there may be some sticking points, blocks, challenges; once you have identified those, reach for a syrupy elixir that is in a vial sitting before you. Breathe deeply and begin to drink the clear, sweet liquid. Let it run through your digestive tract and trap any hint of stress sticking to your gut. The liquid acts like a net, trapping any particulates of impatience, resentment, and burdens. Feel the liquid become absorbed by your gut lining and move into your bloodstream. Watch how the viscous liquid loosens and widens the blood vessel walls, relaxing them so blood can course through your veins and arteries like a quick moving river. Any tightness in your blood vessels dissolves, and the relaxing balm seeps into the blood-vessel walls, making them pliable, flexible, and smooth.

Already, your body has begun to tingle with the delight of becoming alive with the circulation of blood, oxygen, nutrients, and life-force energy. See all four distinct circulation streams running through your body like electrical circuits traveling from head to toe—a red circuit for your blood flow, white for oxygen, green for nutrients, and blue for life-force energy. These circuits weave their ways through every cell, then collectively through every tissue, and, cumulatively, through all organs. Soon after, your entire body is resonating with red, white, green, and blue energy. Breathe in these colors. Relax fully and completely.

The clear viscous liquid that permeated your blood vessels is now ready to be drained from your body. All of it drips down, at its own pace, through the thick of your body tissues and out your feet. From your feet, this liquid saturates the earth below you and trickles through until it finds its way to the earth's core for regeneration.

And now, after the loosening and clearing that has just occurred, say the word *pressure* to yourself once again and see if any residual places in your body respond. For every trace of pressure in your body, actively cancel it and replace it with calm. Use this technique throughout your busy days when you feel overwhelmed; close your eyes, push the cancel button, as if your body were a large computer, and sink into the word *calm*. By practicing this exercise on a daily basis, your blood pressure should begin to respond favorably.

Meditation: Spend about three to five minutes meditating on the word *pressure* and let your mind open to whatever images, words, or thoughts come forth. Keep detached from these responses. Write them down. Now spend the same amount of time meditating on the word *flexibility*, logging any insights or impressions you receive. At the end of the meditation, put together your findings to come up with a solution to make yourself more flexible in the face of pressure.

Blood Pressure, Low (Hypotension)

Physical description: The pressure in blood-vessel walls, in response to the heart pumping blood, is lower than normal, causing reduced blood flow and delivery of oxygen and nutrients to major organs. May result in dizziness, fainting, nausea, and blurred vision.

Energy center(s): Root, heart

Nourishment: *Diet*—(1) Drink adequate water (a general rule of thumb is about eight 8 ounces glasses daily); (2) Refrain from alcohol, as it can be dehydrating; (3) Ensure ingestion of adequate minerals from food sources (e.g., vegetables and vegetable juices, fruits and fruit juices, nuts, sea plants); (4) Ingest moderate amounts of sea salt. *Supplements*—B-complex vitamin containing vitamin B12 and folate.

Emotion(s): Apathy, depression

Limiting belief(s): I lack energy to live life fully. I give up. Living depletes me. The river of life has been drained from me.

Power animal: Elk

Flower essence(s): Buttercup, Cayenne

Affirmation(s): I am motivated to live fully. I am alive! I flow joyously through my days!

Visualization: Envision your body as a collection of instruments, each playing its own sound—the tender violin of the nervous system, the whispering flute of the respiratory system, the pouncing piano of the immune system, the jovial guitar of the musculoskeletal system, the slight percussion of the cardiovascular system. All of them are playing together to make a symphony of sounds, which come together into one musical piece representing your life energy. The only sound that could be strengthened and tweaked is the drumbeat from the heart pumping the blood through the vessels. This part of you has been a bit quiet, and it has resulted in low blood pressure, which causes you to feel off balance from time to time.

Let's tighten up the musical piece by creating a stronger drumbeat. Take deep breaths slowly, and with each one, imagine it changes your blood vessels to be sturdy and stable, yet flexible. From the bottoms of your feet, connect with the pulsating energy of the planet. Let the heartbeat of the earth travel deeply into your bone marrow, its vibration stimulating the marrow to make healthy blood cells. See red blood cells from your bone marrow being sent out to your circulation. They begin populating your blood vessels in healthy numbers.

And, of course, it's important to make sure your body is properly hydrated. Extend your hands out and see all your fingers soaking in streams of crystalline blue water. It courses up your arms, through your neck, and down your torso, hydrating your body. As the water filters in and hydrates you, transform it with the word *invigoration.* Notice how the water crystals take on a beautiful structure that resonates with the energy of *invigoration.* Your body is now saturated, fully hydrated. Your blood cells are healthy and red and travel in the river of the invigorated water.

Visualize the network of blood vessels your body is laced with. See the blood circulating, working together with your blood vessels to bring oxygen and energy to all your tissues.

Go back to the beat of your breath and of the earth, and use this music to propel the circulation of your blood. Let it become loud yet pleasant.

And then, when you feel energized and invigorated, open your inner ears to the music of the other organs. Invite all of the instruments' music to swirl together harmoniously and with the vitality of your life. Envision all the music portrayed as visual shapes and symbols, enveloping you with the music of your life.

Meditation: Find yourself a drum you can beat (it can even be as simple as an aluminum pan). Start drumming slowly and methodically, letting it gradually become stronger and faster paced. Imagine the drumbeat is a metaphor for the rhythmic flow of your blood.

Bone Healing (Fracture or Break)

Physical description: A bone breaks due to mechanical stress or force.

Energy center(s): Root

Nourishment: *Diet*—(1) Reduce animal products (meats, cheeses) and eliminate caffeinated drinks; (2) Eat copious amounts of alkalizing (high in potassium) fresh vegetables (especially green ones) to help the body to establish optimal pH for bone healing. *Supplements*—(1) Vitamin C and bioflavonoids for rebuilding the collagen matrix of bone; (2) Vitamin K for healthy formation of bone proteins; (3) Arnica homeopathic remedy for trauma; (4) A multimineral supplement (including calcium, magnesium, and zinc).

Emotion(s): Insecurity, feeling unsupported

Limiting belief(s): My inner and outer security is fragile and broken. My life has come crashing down on me. I lack support. I am unable to stand up for myself. I am overburdened.

Power animal: Beaver

Flower essence(s): Arnica, Echinacea, Sweet Pea

Affirmation(s): I am fully supported and strong. I am stable and secure in myself.

Visualization: Imagine your feet are like mineral magnets, and they pull up from the earth's crust any minerals your bones need for healing of cracks or breaks. Give yourself a couple of seconds so these minerals can find their way to your feet. See a mass of minerals, like clusters, collecting and forming at the bottom of your feet. Your feet feel heavy and weighted down by their strong pull. When you are ready, use your inhaled breath to reach down into these masses, and then with your exhale, move the minerals through your whole skeleton—through all the tiny bones in the feet, ankles, legs, pelvis, spine, ribs, shoulders, arms, and hands, and up into the skull. Take your time in doing this and ensure that every single inch of bony space in your body has been filled in and dense with the minerals from the earth. Wherever you may have your break or fracture, provide extra minerals to the bony matrix there. Make sure it feels strong with minerals, yet still pliable and movable.

In your mind's eye, see your skeleton as a glowing white outline, almost electric, with sufficient energy to balance the bone-forming and bone-breakdown cells. You feel supported by your skeleton.

Now imagine you pull in through your feet another type of energy. This time, it's the warm, loving, supportive healing energy contained within the earth—the energy that courses through the entire planet like blood in veins. This nurturing, red, warm energy glides through your feet and fluidly flows upwards, circling around your tailbone and pelvis, to give you unconditional support in your attempts to survive in the physical world. This energy replaces any stuck financial stress or any fears about survival and security. It moves its way into your low belly and up into your heart area, saturating you with emotional support and balance in your ability to give and receive. It spirals upward into your shoulders to throw off any burdens about having to support others. You are relieved from all back-breaking stress in your life; it has been washed out and replaced by love and support of a high quality.

When you are finished washing the nurturing, healing energy of the earth through your body, notice how every other part in your body now supports your skeleton, in addition to your skeleton supporting your body by providing the body's frame.

Meditation: Meditate on the area of fracture being infused with green healing light that pours forth from your heart. As you do this, reflect on all the ways in your life you are supported.

Breast Problems (Cysts, Lumps, Soreness)

Physical description: Breast growths, such as cysts and lumps, can range from being a benign (noncancerous), fluid-filled sac (a soft or firm round or oval lump) to cancerous growths. Tenderness can occur in the area of the growth. It is thought that excess estrogen plays a role in their development.

Energy center(s): Sacral, heart

Nourishment: *Diet*—(1) Eat foods high in phytoestrogens ("plant estrogens," which are weaker sources of estrogen that can block the activity of biological estrogen in the body), such as legumes (lentils, garbanzo beans, whole soybeans, black beans), whole grains (whole-grain breads and cereals, flaxseed meal, oat bran), and vegetables; (Please note that phytoestrogens are considered mildly estrogenic and may not be suitable for individuals with hormone-sensitive cancers. Check with your healthcare professional as to whether phytoestrogen-containing foods would be appropriate for you.) (2) Eat high-fiber foods, such as berries (blackberries and raspberries are best), pears and apples with the skin, whole grains like cooked barley or bran flakes, cooked legumes (split peas and lentils), peas, broccoli, and brussels sprouts; (3) Eat high-sulfur foods such as garlic and onion. *Supplements*—Fiber supplements such as pectin, guar gum, ground flaxseed meal, or psyllium.

Emotion(s): Inadequacy, buried anger, hurt

Limiting belief(s): I value others more than myself. My needs are unimportant. Nurturing myself feels selfish. I must protect others, even if it means neglecting myself. It is my responsibility to protect and care for others.

Power animal: Hawk

Flower essence(s): Alpine Lily, Mariposa Lily, Pink Yarrow

Affirmation(s): I nurture my self. My femininity is in balance. I form healthy boundaries between myself and others. My ability to nourish and my need for nourishment are perfectly balanced.

Visualization: Close your eyes and put your awareness into the center of your chest. Examine the three-dimensional landscape unfolding before you. Make yourself small and begin to tour the area of your heart, walking through all of its magnificent caverns and tunnels and observing the strong, passionate beat moving blood through your body.

And then take a journey into your lungs, diving into the fine layers of your lung tissue with the inhale of your breath and bouncing out again with the exhale. Notice the distinct rhythms of your body, your heart and your lungs chiming together in harmony.

Your body has its own unique sound that you hum to. Tune into the beauty of its beat. Lose your awareness to its mystery, engulfing yourself in it, bathing your consciousness in it, as if it were surround-stereo sound. It is you, yet you are observing it while being neutral at the same time. While you are listening to your rhythm, let it turn into a visual image—a rolling ribbon of silky, shimmering silver and gold. As the music plays, the ribbon dances along, matching the tunes.

With a strong beat of the heart, or with an inhale or exhale of the lungs, the ribbon dances upward and in a spiral motion. In the absence of the heartbeat or in the between stages of a breath, it moves freely through space. You guide the ribbon, your beat, with your intention. The dancing cosmos within you has the ability to heal you, if that is your intent.

Swirl two colors of the ribbon together, the liquid light of silver and gold, and swish the combined form through the inner cavity and tissue of both of your breasts. Fill them completely with the liquid light so there is no room for any darkness, shadows, cysts, lumps, soreness, pain. Any and all of those things, if they are present, dissolve and transform into the glittery light.

Circulate and spin the ribbon of light at a slow speed within both breasts. Gradually accelerate it to medium speed and, finally, to a high speed for just a couple of seconds. The light purifies, cleanses, and strengthens the breast tissue. When it has accomplished what it has needed to do, let it exit through your nipples and pour into an empty glass in front of you.

Feel an opening throughout your chest, expanding wide and far, like an entire expanse of grassy meadow dotted with millions of wildflowers. See yourself dancing freely through this field with your arms open wide, embracing the fresh air surrounding you and taking in the aroma of field flowers into every pore of your skin.

When you feel energized, open, and liberated, lie down in the grass, spreading your body like a starfish. Visualize your pulsing heart-lung-breast energy as a spiraling disc of green light in the center of your chest. This light begins to radiate out through all six lanes of your body—through your head, two arms, two legs, and tailbone. You are a radiating emerald star, at one with nature, giving forth your glow of life.

And now, after you have given of your energy to the planet, let the planet feed its energy through you so that you may be nourished. Draw energy—the cumulative swirling energy of the moon, stars, sun, planets, sky, and universe—into all six limbs of your body. Pull in this tremendous energy and have all paths coalesce in the heart-lung-breast region. Sit with this energy for a couple of seconds, and let it nourish you completely. Be fed by all of life.

When you feel ready, visualize yourself in a standing position, with the glass of radiant, shining gold-silver liquid light before you. See how it sparkles, shines, and beams forth. Pour this liquid light down over you, starting from your head and allowing it to cascade down your body, through every pore, chakra, cell, meridian, and subtle body. You are engulfed in nourishing radiance. When you feel ready, invite yourself to slowly release the visualization. Mentally affirm, "My ability to nourish and my need for nourishment are perfectly balanced."

Meditation: Spend at least five minutes per day doing what *you*'d like to do. If you are unsure of what those activities could be, try meditating on possibilities.

Bulimia

Physical description: A condition marked by episodes of binge eating (defined as eating excessively during one sitting and feeling out of control) followed by a compensatory behavior, such as self-induced vomiting, overexercising, fasting, or using laxatives, enemas, and/or diuretics.

Energy center(s): Root, solar plexus, throat, third eye

Nourishment: *Diet*—Begin a practice of mindful eating by taking time to eat. Note your level of fullness after each meal, rating it on scale of one to ten.

Emotion(s): Feeling overwhelmed, feeling unfulfilled, regret, hurt

Limiting belief(s): I can never get enough to satisfy me. My life leaves me hungry for more. I crave fulfillment. I stuff down my emotions and release them under controlled situations. I've got to be perfect to be satisfied.

Power animal: Lizard

Flower essence(s): Beech, Chicory

Affirmation(s): I am fulfilled. Life nourishes me inside and out. Perfection lies within the seeming imperfection.

Visualization: Imagine that before you lays a feast, only instead of it consisting of foods you know and love to eat, it is composed of different items. In one bowl, you see not salad, but a medley of leaves of grace, seeds of abundance, coated with a dressing of forgiveness. The colorful array of fruits and vegetables is a symbol of balance and prosperity. The main course is unconditional love, served over and over again on skewers. For dessert, there is a bowl not of ice cream, but of pure sweetness and joy. Indulge in the qualities these foods bring forth, taking samplings of the grace, abundance, and forgiveness. Bite into them and even devour them voraciously. Chew thoroughly to maximize everything you can take in.

And then shift your palate to the artist's palette of colors created by the array of fruits and vegetables. Take in all the different colors, filling up on the stability of red, the creativity of orange, the power of yellow, the love of green, the truth of blue, the mystery of indigo, and the purity of white. Swirl them all together in your mouth and swallow this essence.

For the main course, dive in to the unconditional love, eating it with your hands, getting right into the thick of it. Fill yourself with the amazement of what it feels like to be loved and to give love.

Finally, indulge in the pure sweetness of joy by taking as many spoonfuls of this creamy fun as you need.

When you are finished with this bountiful feast, sit back and relax. Invite these beautiful flavors, tastes, and nourishment you have taken in to find their place within the onionlike layers of yourself, including your physical body, emotional body, intellectual body, and spiritual body. See them all settling into place, creating flow and harmony within all your layers by establishing a network between them all.

After you have given yourself a couple of seconds or even minutes to let yourself digest this experience, you are now ready to release anything and everything within your consciousness that provides a barrier to your full potential. Allow a couple of seconds for these barriers to come forth and then move them out of your body, through your mouth, the pores of your skin, and out your feet. Clear your entire being of self-betrayal, guilt, control, fear, and anger, making room for all the empowering qualities that you just took in. See streams of these barriers flushing out of your system.

And when you feel you have cleared them from your being, come back fully into the present moment. Sit at the table that held the feast earlier. You have eaten all foods of high-consciousness qualities, and all the plates and bowls have been cleared away. A dazzling array of flowers sits in a vase in front of you. You take in their sweet smell and open your eyes to your new self.

Meditation: Spend one meal per day eating mindfully, dedicated to your inner fulfillment on physical, emotional, mental, and spiritual levels.

Bunions (SEE FOOT PAIN)

Cancer

Physical description: Uncontrolled cell growth resulting in organ dysfunction.

Energy center(s): Sacral (Depending on where the cancer is located, other chakras may be involved. For instance, prostate cancer connects to the root chakra.)

Nourishment: *Diet*—(1) Refrain from eating overly processed, high-sugar, high-fat foods, and reduce sodium; (2) Shift from eating animal fat (saturated fat) and protein (like smoked and cured meats) to eating primarily vegetables and whole grains; (3) Emphasize vegetables with detoxifying properties, such as broccoli, cabbage, brussels sprouts, onions, and garlic, as well as colorful vegetables in every area of the spectrum—red vegetables rich in lycopene, such as tomatoes and beets; orange vegetables high in beta-carotene, such as pumpkin and carrots; green-yellow vegetables high in lutein, like spinach and leeks; (4) Drink teas made from any of the following: pau d'arco, burdock, and dandelion; (5) Favor organically grown food over conventionally produced.

Emotion(s): Hurt, self-containment, self-suppression, fear

Limiting belief(s): I am out of control. My hurtful feelings have proliferated. I am taken over by unexpressed creativity. My wounds are buried in my body. It's dangerous to express my true self creatively. I refuse my creative ability.

Power animal: Lamb

Flower essence(s): Black-eyed Susan, Echinacea, Willow

Affirmation(s): I see everything as perfect. My feelings are creatively expressed. My body follows a healthy process of beginnings and ends. I embrace my ability to create.

Visualization: *It would be preferable if you can find a way to lie down to in order to relax.*

Imagine your body is lying in between two panels of durable material. These panels are held up in space and are stacked one on top of the other, with about four feet in between them. The sides of the panels facing you are shiny silver, and the exteriors, facing away from you, are porcelain white.

Your body rests between them, like the filling of a sandwich, although you are not stuffed or cramped, and you actually feel comfortable and warm within the embrace of these two panels. Take an easy inhale to adjust yourself within this enclosed structure. Make sure you feel calm. Have your arms at your sides; your feet are relaxed, and your eyes are closed.

These panels have the ability to generate healing light. As you go through this visualization, a series of colored lights will be scanning your body, altering your cellular composition and genetic material. Like the light of a scanner or copier, the lights will start in one place and travel to the next. Each scanning light will move from the top of your head to the bottom of your feet, and then the next one will start. The lights will be strengthening your body's defenses and releasing any dead or cancerous cells. Take your time going through each of the healing lights. When you feel ready, wiggle your toes and begin the visualization.

The first light to come through is a deep, rich red. The deep red light will detect in your body or energy field any misalignment of the DNA within your cells. Any damaged or mutated DNA will be repaired by this moving red light. It will dissolve any bacteria, fungi, or virus inconsistent with your good health. Its nourishing light also invigorates the blood and gets your circulation moving with increasing speed and without obstruction. Your immune system becomes fed by this red light. Let it course through the entire extent of your body, cleansing your physical body and making way for healing to occur.

The next light to come through is a bright orange light—the color of the insides of a papaya. Soft and lingering, it starts at your head and moves slowly down to your feet, picking up, like a magnet, any residual emotional patterns trapped within your cells. Your emotional body begins to feel free and flowing as all stagnant emotions are released. You feel an immediate clearing, and your creative juices are flowing in a rhythm perfect for your body. Your cells are aligned with abundant, yet balanced, creativity, and the cycles of growth within the cells are now becoming regulated, defined, and healthy.

The next light to come through is a brilliant, dazzling yellow, as bright as the sun. It makes its way from head to toe in a zigzag fashion, infusing you with stamina, esteem, and power. Each cell in your body becomes revved by the presence of this miraculous yellow light. All the energy-making machinery in your body is cleared of any gunk. At once, you *feel* light and energized. Your body is in perfect energy balance, giving out the right amount of energy and taking in a balanced amount of energy. Your digestive system is renewed with the sunlight energy, using the fire element to transform anything its way to what can be of use for your body.

The yellow light is followed by a rich emerald glow, similar to the color of an actual emerald or of a lush, green forest. It carries the energy of unconditional love, acceptance, and nurturing and moves through your body as though your body were a garden being sprinkled with fertilizer, water, and sunlight. You are nourished at a profound level by the presence of the emerald glow. It permeates your mind, the area around your heart, your torso, and your pelvis, and then moves out through your legs and feet. Anything not having heart is removed and shuffled out. You feel an aliveness wash over you.

In an instant, the green glow is followed up by a soothing aquamarine light the same color as a summer sky. It engulfs every part of you, slowly and completely. Its infusion becomes alchemy in your body. Your physical, emotional, mental, and spiritual bodies become shiny gold, imbued with your sense of truth and authenticity. Words remaining unexpressed, or words or actions that have left impressions on you in a negative way, continuing to live with you, are expelled forth into the aquamarine light, like clouds floating in the sky. Your throat and mouth feel more open; your body feels free to express and create in a way conducive to who you are.

Next, a potent indigo-violet light, vibrating at a rapid rate, enters. It carries so much healing and depth that it is able to slice right through you, moving slowly and stopping at places that need additional assistance. This light brings to you insight and wisdom, and helps you to reanimate your sense of imagination. Your cells swirl with delight as they are bathed in its presence. This light carries the essence of protection to your many layers.

And, finally, a blinding white light glides evenly over your entire body to end the session. It has the energy of a diamond, with many facets and high value. Every photon of this light dances within your core and touches each cell, and by the time the light reaches your feet, your cells are interconnected and harmonized by the white light.

Take a generous deep breath. You may go back and re-run any of the lights you feel necessary. When you are ready, wiggle your toes, which will allow the two panels to dissipate into the ethers, and you will be left comfortably in your resting position. Open your eyes and observe how healthy, clean, cleared, and harmonized your body feels.

Meditation: Draw an outline of your body. Meditate on the areas that feel stuck or stagnant, or that are accumulating energy. Mark them on your drawing. Meditate on how to relieve these areas of the body. Welcome the solutions you are presented with.

Candida Albicans, Overgrowth (SEE YEAST INFECTION)

Carpal Tunnel Syndrome

Physical description: A painful, tingling, burning, or numb and weak sensation in the fingers due to compression of the median nerve running from the forearm into the hand at the level of the wrist. Typically found in those who engage in repetitive work with their hands.

Energy center(s): Heart, crown

Nourishment: *Diet*—Eat more foods rich in vitamin B6, such as leafy, green vegetables; nuts; legumes; cabbage; bananas; and cantaloupe, to name a few.

Emotion(s): Irritation, burning anger, helplessness

Limiting belief(s): I am angry for feeling helpless. I am numb to my personal expression. My heart's passion is unable to be expressed. My life is mundane.

Power animal: Otter

Flower essence(s): California Wild Rose, Indian Paintbrush, Iris

Affirmation(s): I am insightful about how to express myself. I liberate my passions through my work. My hands give and receive equally.

Visualization: Gently and carefully, raise your arms in front of you and rotate your wrists simultaneously in a clockwise direction. With your subtle movement, unlock any stored energy or blocks that have become a part of your delicate wrists. Visualize green-blue light coming through your shoulders, arms, and wrists and out through your hands as you do this. Ask yourself, what do I feel I can no longer provide or give? Wait for your answer.

And now let your arms drop to their respective sides of your body. Close your eyes while you either stand or sit in a relaxed manner.

Tune in to the energy of your heart. Imagine you have a key that opens the door of your heart, allowing you inside of it. As the door opens, a rush of emerald green energy of love pours forth. Let the energy of love cascade down your shoulders and arms like a gushing waterfall. The force of the energy coursing through your arms releases them of all stored tension. All the nerves are liberated and freed from an obstruction. The muscles soften. Your bones are nourished by the flow. Any pain from overwork or from a constant giving of your energy is balanced by your receptivity of this flow of love. The green cascade circles through your wrists and then radiates out of every finger on both hands. Your chest and arms expand and release their tightness.

A beautiful angel then gives you two bracelets to wear on your wrists. The one for the left wrist is silver and embodies the energy of the moon, the ability to receive and create. The one for the right wrist is gold and carries within its smooth band the energy of the sun, or the inclination to act and grow. You slip the bracelets on, and your wrists begin to tingle with the infusion of energy. The two wrists are connected to one another through invisible lines of magnetism generated by the energetic bracelets. Each one supports the other.

And now, come to a close by resuming your initial wrist-motion exercise, keeping your arms outstretched before you and moving your wrists—this time back and forth and from side to side. Feel the lightness inside them, and mentally affirm, "I give and receive equally."

Meditation: Meditate for a couple of minutes with your fingers in a specific mudra, or hand position, that connects your fiery, creative expression to your ability to be grounded in everyday life. Turn your palms upward and touch the tip of each middle finger to the tip of the thumb on the same hand. Sit comfortably while you meditate on fire and earth energies circulating through your body in harmony.

Celiac Disease

Physical description: The inability to tolerate the ingestion of dietary gluten (a protein commonly found in barley, rye, wheat, and spelt), resulting in small-intestine damage that can lead to diarrhea, weight loss, infertility, nutrient deficiencies, nausea, bloating, anemia, skin rash, and joint/bone pain, to name a few symptoms.

Energy center(s): Sacral, solar plexus

Nourishment: *Diet*—(1) Avoid all gluten-containing foods by abstaining from products containing wheat, barley, rye, oat, and spelt. Corn and rice are good substitutes for these grains. Read labels carefully, as many additives are derived from gluten-containing ingredients (e.g., wheat-derived maltodextrin, hydrolyzed wheat protein); (2) Reduce or eliminate dairy products, as individuals who are gluten intolerant tend to be intolerant of other proteins, specifically dairy-derived proteins; (3) Exercise caution in eating too many gluten-free processed foods (e.g., cookies, bagels, breads), as they tend to be high in refined sugar; (4) Emphasize high-fiber, fresh foods like vegetables, legumes, seeds, nuts, and fruits; (5) Investigate food allergies and nutrient deficiencies with the help of a qualified healthcare professional. *Supplements*—(1) High-potency multivitamin (with a complete spectrum of B vitamins); (2) Probiotics for establishing better gut health; (3) Pancreatic enzymes for enhancing nutrient digestion; (4) Omega-3 oil supplement (fish or flaxseed oil) for reducing inflammation.

Emotion(s): Insecurity, vulnerability, feeling overwhelmed, feeling unable to "take it all in"—especially with regard to issues involving family, security, and safety

Limiting belief(s): I am unable to process life. There is resistance in what I am willing to take in. I am overwhelmed with insecurity. I haven't accomplished anything. I am worn down.

Power animal: Goat

Flower essence(s): California Poppy, Cerato, Dill, Sweet Pea

Affirmation(s): I integrate and synthesize my life events. I feel safe in my gut. I am accomplished. I process life with love, creativity, and expression.

Visualization: Close your eyes and drop your attention to your gut at the level of your navel. Out of your navel, imagine your gut unwinds itself out of your body; a several-feet-long tube presents itself before you. See if there are any hurts locked within or stuck to your gut. Envision running a narrow tube of white-and-pink light through it, saturating it to the extent that your intestines begin to take on a warm glow on the outside. Imagine this white-and-pink light feeds your gut exactly what it needs and takes away what is no longer needed. It stimulates the enzymes in your gut to break down gluten. It helps to seal the gut wall so it is not leaky. It even helps to recharge the small fingerlike structures (called villi) lining the gut, making them receptive to nutrients.

This healing, healthy light is the ultimate nourishment for your intestines. You always have access to this healing power, and one way to use it is to combine your foods with it as they travel down your gut when you eat.

Now, as your intestines soak in this light, gaze at them lovingly, sending compassion and kindness through your internal eyes. Give your intestines the freedom and ability to be creative by forming shapes before you—perhaps shapes that are relevant to what you need more of in your life, or healing forms specifically for you. Let your gut move without resistance and dance its way around you. What does it say? What does it feel? What creative impulses are infusing you? Savor the feeling of being liberated and the wonderful state of being acquainted with your gut, which you have not known like this before.

When you have received the information you feel is necessary at this time, with your intention, guide your gut, now filled with healing light and basking in your love and acceptance, back into your body through your navel center. Let it coil in comfortably, snuggling inside, feeling warm, cared for, and fully expressive. Affirm to your gut, "I process life with love, creativity, and expression."

Meditation: For a whole week, practice allowing your gut to lead the way. Before making decisions, feel the response in your gut area. See how often you are able to honor your gut, what you feel after doing so, and what you feel after not listening to it.

Chlamydia (SEE VENEREAL DISEASE)

Common Cold

Physical description: A viral infection in the upper respiratory tract, resulting in head and sinus congestion, fatigue, coughing, headache, fever, the inability to sleep, and overall body aches.

Energy center(s): Root, heart, throat

Nourishment: *Diet*—(1) Drink adequate fluids, including warm broths (e.g., vegetable, chicken, turkey) and teas (herbal teas are best: echinacea, pau d'arco, ginger, chamomile); (2) Avoid all sugar-containing foods, as they depress immune system function. *Supplements*—(1) Vitamin C and bioflavonoids for reducing the duration of the cold; (2) Zinc lozenges for a healthy immune system; (3) *Echinacea purpurea* root (as dry root, juice, tincture, or extract) to help strengthen the immune system and reduce cold duration.

Emotion(s): Feeling invaded, feeling overwhelmed

Limiting belief(s): Overwork is necessary. I take it all in. My value rests in how much I do. I can never do enough.

Power animal: Porcupine

Flower essence(s): Beech, Centaury, Clematis, Hornbeam, Oak

Affirmation(s): I know what is me and not me. I am protected and secure in my self. I am worthy.

Visualization: *Practice this visualization the moment you feel susceptible to a cold coming on and frequently throughout the days you are healing from the infection.*

Release yourself fully into the moment. Collect all of your pieces—physical, emotional, mental, and spiritual—and assemble them together so you feel them and can see them more clearly.

Put the tip of your tongue to the roof of your mouth, ever so slightly, and take yourself into the center of your head. With your gaze going inward, find yourself at precisely the point at which two lines traveling from the ears inward and from the top of the head down would intersect. Keep your consciousness here, fully and completely, and notice whether you sense or see an image. Is this space clear? Or is it full of mist and clouds? What obstructions do you see? What thought patterns are swirling in this area? Take your time gathering in the essence of this space, so you know it fully.

Breathe into this space. Carry your breath up and into your head, clearing any images, blocks, thoughts, and patterns that no longer serve you. Let them all collect in one place, and with a full exhale, move them from your being. Try this three more times: breathe in to your head space even more breath, if you can; swirl it around in your inner head, where it acts as a whirlpool to get together things that are inconsistent with your life's purpose—whether those things are images of people, daily activities, undue stress, piles of responsibilities, worry, lack of boundaries; and allow these things to funnel out of you, either through your nostrils or through your mouth.

The third time you are breathing in, soft, healing, golden light fills your headspace, illuminating any crevices, corners, or uncharted territory from the previous breaths. Like a shining light in the dark, this light uncovers anything not already been brought forth. And into the light steps any situations or limiting beliefs connected to your self-worth, your identity, or your ability to achieve and perform. The light makes any issues hiding in your subconscious very apparent. With your next exhale, show them the way out of your body. Bless and release them and ask that you may replace these parts in your mind with thoughts of love and self-acceptance.

At this time, imagine you take in an elixir of breath, which rushes through your whole body and penetrates your bone marrow, your thymus, and your white blood cells, giving them the strength and energy they need to ward off any remaining physical effects of out-side invaders, including microbes, viruses, fungi, or parasites. Invaders that are no longer welcome parade out of your body through your subsequent exhales. Your body feels full of energy and, at the same time, peace. This feeling extends around your body about seven feet.

When you are ready, move slowly into your life routine, savoring additional rest and liquids, and remembering that you are clear and supported from within.

Meditation: Notice in your interactions with people how you feel nourished by some individuals and depleted, and even emotionally drained, by others. Become aware of this sensation and meditate on how you can come up with solutions to create better boundaries when you are confronted with a draining, invasive situation or event.

Constipation

Physical description: Infrequent or difficult bowel movements

Energy center(s): Root, sacral

Nourishment: *Diet*—(1) Drink adequate water on a daily basis (about eight 8-oz. glasses, half your body weight in ounces, or the smaller of the two); (2) Eat high-fiber foods, like legumes, vegetables, berries, nuts, seeds, and ground flaxseed meal; (3) Reduce your intake of animal-derived foods, such as meats and dairy products; (4) Eat when you are relaxed rather than on the run; (5) Ensure that you are getting enough oils (e.g., olive oil, flaxseed oil, fish oil), aiming for about four teaspoons per day. *Supplements*—(1) Fiber supplement (e.g., oat bran, pectin, guar gum, psyllium); (2) Occasional, moderate use of Aloe vera juice can be moistening as well as cooling for the gut; (3) Vitamin C (about 1 gram daily, in separate doses) and magnesium (about 400 mg daily) act as natural laxatives; use with caution, preferably under the supervision of a healthcare professional, and only for the short term.

Emotion(s): Untrusting, fear

Limiting belief(s): If I hold it in, I won't hurt anybody. Letting go only means pain. I cling to the past for fear of the future.

Power animal: Wolf

Flower essence(s): Angel's Trumpet, Blackberry, Walnut

Affirmation(s): I flow forward. I release stuck energy to make way for new, invigorating energy. I surrender.

Visualization: Let your childlike imagination run free and use it to transpose your body into the image of a landscape—a desert. See your body before you as miles and miles of dry, parched land, soaking in the sunrays, but longing for moisture and replenishment. Let your awareness be embodied by a small person traversing the seemingly endless span of crisp, cracked land. Feel yourself blanketed by the strong heat of the sunrays. Are there any objects on this landscape capturing your attention? If so, let yourself interact with them. Gather any information they are willing to share.

When you are ready, allow this body landscape of yours to transform into the opposite of the desert—a lush forested area. Step back, as if you were an artist, and command objects and scenery into your body space. Start with the area close to your head and invite in a garden of fruit trees, where the fruit hangs ripe, like newfound ideas. Through the neck, see the flow of a strong large river. It flows upwards from the delta of the heart. Envision that you see words, passion, ideas as being fluid, moving up from the heart and into the hearty rush of the river in the throat and coursing out of the mouth. Circulate small pools of water in each of the shoulders, relieving any burdens and dissolving them into the water, so they are released and moved out of the body via the river.

The river is lined with fertile ground all around it. As you make your way into your torso, see your gut area as the most fertile, lush jungle possible. Fill it with large tropical trees growing fruits like bananas and coconuts. See clear, trickling streams lacing their way through your intestines, moisturizing the dried space that was deserted just moments ago. Your intestines are lubricated with the sparkling water coursing through them. Any barrier or stuck feeling, like a rock in the fast-moving stream, becomes worn away by the flow of the water until it has completely disappeared. Feel the tightness and constriction, the feeling of holding back, dissolve into the cascading water. The vibration of the current ripples through the caverns of your internal organs, massaging and infusing them with relaxation, surrender, and peace.

Inside the hollow of your legs, long, swinging vines anchor themselves into the soil beneath your feet. Any resistance felt in your lower body makes its way out by climbing down your legs and exiting out of your feet, and then it sinks into the loamy earth.

Your body has completely morphed from being dry, parched, and thirsty for expression into one that is moist, healing, lush, and animated with the expression of your being.

Meditation: Become aware of at least one thing in your life that would be beneficial to let go of. Reflect on one aspect you would welcome into your space in the place of what you need to release.

Coughing

Physical description: An involuntary or voluntary reflex of keeping the throat and airways clear by forcing air out of the lungs in an effort to expel excessive secretions, irritants, and/or particles.

Energy center(s): Heart, throat

Nourishment: Keep throat lubricated with adequate warm liquids, such as tea (licorice, marshmallow) and water (with lemon). Try lozenges made from slippery elm.

Emotion(s): Conflict, internal and external. Moist cough—expulsion of buried grief. Dry, crackling, forced cough—expression of built-up anger, brittleness, and wanting to be noticed and acknowledged.

Limiting belief(s): I am less than. I harbor my pain inside. My feelings want to be noticed. I hold back from saying how I really feel.

Power animal: Owl

Flower essence(s): Black-eyed Susan, Chamomile, Echinacea, Yerba Santa

Affirmation(s): I believe in myself. I speak my truth if I feel called. I am a conduit of grace and light. I speak my truth loud and clear.

Visualization: Sink your attention into the back of your throat and let it glide down your throat, coating your throat like a lozenge. Be here for a thick moment. The throat is a tube of expression for your heart, which includes all your feelings, passions, wisdom, and experience. Is there anything within your throat preventing you from the expression of your heart? Is there any lodged fear, resentment, bitterness, lack of joy, or anger sitting nestled in your throat space? If so, let them fly out like bats escaping from a cave, being liberated and in the light of day. No more darkness, shadows, or unfelt emotions line your throat. Imagine it as a shaft of brilliant blue light, serving as a conduit or a vessel of communication. Any words not expelled will be put into small boxes and shipped out of your throat.

Imagine an elixir of truth sitting in an intricate vial before you. Drink from this vial, and let it coat the inside of your mouth and the expanse of your throat. This elixir is so powerful that it saturates the entire lining of your mucous membranes, extending even up into your sinuses, and heals them with the presence of your inner truth. It dries up any excess mucous and rebalances the water and earth element within this region of your body. It is your authenticity that heals your coughing; your need to speak up and get attention on something that is important to you.

As the elixir travels down into your being, it slowly blankets your body in an inner layer of protection to shield you from invading viruses, bacteria, or any other microorganisms. It also traps any lingering microorganisms that are not beneficial and true for you; it coats and immobilizes them.

With the consistency of honey, the elixir winds its way down your body until it drizzles its way out your feet and into the healing confines of the earth. The earth absorbs this truth, and as it does so, it becomes more liquefied until it turns into water, then mist, and then air.

With a long breath in, you breathe in your truth so it fills every molecule of your being. This fresh air clears your body of any debris or block that may cause you to cough. Your lungs are energized and clear. Think of this breath every time you feel the need to cough. Speak aloud, "I speak my truth loud and clear."

Meditation: Write down all the things you'd like to say, but have not yet said.

Depression

Physical description: An overall feeling of sadness, worthlessness, or being disinterested in life events to the extent that it interferes with everyday life. Other symptoms include excessive sleeping, changes in appetite, and body aches.

Energy center(s): Root, third eye, crown

Nourishment: *Diet*—(1) Balance blood sugar by eating foods that have low-glycemic-index ratings, such as legumes, vegetables (non-starchy), lean protein, fruits (except ripe bananas), low-fat dairy, and whole grains; (2) Eat foods high in omega-3 fats, such as fish, leafy greens, nuts, and seeds. *Supplements*—(1) Omega-3 fatty-acid supplement (fish or flaxseed oil) to promote healthy fat deposition in brain; (2) B-complex vitamin to provide cofactors needed for neurotransmitter synthesis; (3) St. John's wort to improve mood, and decrease anxiety and insomnia (Note: Use under supervision of healthcare professional if you are taking other supplements or drugs.); (4) 5-hydroxytryptophan (5-HTP) to improve mood.

Emotion(s): Anger, rage, loneliness, feeling disconnected from life

Limiting belief(s): I am isolated and separate. I lack connection with a greater purpose. I have let myself and others down. I have failed.

Power animal: Ant

Flower essence(s): Mustard, Sweet Chestnut, White Chestnut, Wild Oat

Affirmation(s): At all times, I am connected with my highest potential. My life is filled with the light of possibilities and opportunities. I welcome my life's purpose.

Visualization: Plant your feet firmly on the earth. Let your entire awareness sink down into the soles of your feet until you begin to feel the heartbeat of the planet resonating in the four corners of your feet.

Feel her aliveness, her strength, in the rhythm of this incessant beat. It begins to awaken you on a deep level.

Allow the pulsing of the earth to travel up your legs, stabilizing them. At the same time, this active percussion sound tickles every cell of your lower body. Zoom in to the level of your cells and see their lightness and laughter at this infusion of earth energy. They begin to chatter and send messages back and forth between neighboring cells.

Let the pulsing find its home at the base of your spine, like a soothing, nourishing drumbeat on your low back. This rhythm wakes up in you any part that is asleep and dormant to all of life. It connects you to the web of nature—the trees, the sky, the grass, all animals, and all humans. And in an instant, you feel invigorated. You are imbued with the right to exist. The mission of living circulates freely and rapidly through your bloodstream. It pulses within you, shaking out any negativity, stagnation, blocks, or challenges, transforming and dispersing them, like fertilizer to your entire being, and giving you an added electrical current running through your spine and through the wiring of your nervous system. The branches of your nervous system become electrified with earth energy, and the feeling of aliveness ripples through your brain, changing the activity of your neurotransmitters in a beneficial way.

From your brain, the energy of life shoots down your spinal column, and from the nerves, that network through the spine, all organ systems become invigorated. Your hands, head, heart, gut, and low back accumulate this energy for a couple of seconds and then send it back to the earth in separate streams of electric blue. The earth energy continues to feed in through your feet, and a circulation of energy back to the earth occurs once again after this energy has run through you and fed you with healing, positive messages of living.

Continue to vision this cycle as many times as you need.

Meditation: Find a cause you care deeply about. Make a commitment to its purpose by volunteering, donating resources, or simply sending a note of gratitude.

Diabetes (See Hyperglycemia)

Diarrhea

Physical description: Frequent, loose watery stools.

Energy center(s): Root, sacral

Nourishment: *Diet*—(1) Replenish fluids and electrolytes by drinking liquids such as fresh fruit and vegetable juices; (2) Eat high-fiber foods (e.g., beans, berries, nonstarchy vegetables like spinach) to promote bulky stools; (3) Work with a qualified healthcare professional to identify food allergies. *Supplements*—(1) Probiotics (e.g., *Lactobacillus rhamnosus, Lactobacillus GG)* to help reestablish healthy gut flora; (2) A fiber supplement (e.g., psyllium, pectin, guar gum, oat fiber) to promote bulking.

Emotion(s): Extremes of emotions, emotional exhaustion, emptiness, turbulence

Limiting belief(s): I live by unhealthy extremes. I feel out of control. An emptiness fills me. I always feel on alert, unable to live my life comfortably.

Power animal: Dolphin

Flower essence(s): Black Cohosh, Dogwood, Morning Glory

Affirmation(s): I am flowing with the rhythm of life at my own pace. I move with peace. I am filled with harmony.

Visualization: Imagine you are gifted with an energetic vacuum cleaner that has the ability to draw from you that which you do not need. The vacuum can shrink and expand as required by the task. You shrink the vacuum so it is small enough to fit in your mouth, and you swallow it, moving it through using the peristaltic rhythm of your gut until it gets to your large intestine.

In the large intestine, there is a bit more room, and so you enlarge the vacuum a bit more. You set it into motion, soaking up all the excess water. This energetic vacuum has unlimited storage and, as a result, can draw in as much water as is needed in order to bring your bowel movements back to normal. Give the vacuum a couple of seconds to make its way through the long, tunnel-like structure of the large intestine. In addition to excess water, the vacuum can extract any energetic debris, microorganisms, or toxins that cause the colon to be imbalanced. Visualize this cleansing and drying taking place very systematically through the stretch of the intestine until, finally, the vacuum cleaner is done with its job and exits your gut. Already, you feel much more balanced and full of energy than before.

The next step is to replenish your gut with healthy bacteria to keep out pathogenic invaders. Envision in your hand a capsule containing all the healthy bacteria you need to repopulate your gut. Swallow the capsule, mentally following it down to your lower intestine, where the contents are allowed to disperse throughout the gut. See the bacteria adhering on to the intestinal wall, providing security and protection.

Finally, you see two separate vials of liquid in front of you. In the first one is an opaque, glossy liquid of a vibrant, healthy orange color, like the color of a sunset. You drink it in, and the contents quickly meander down to your colon, coating the colon with its radiance. It creates a strong layer in the inner wall of the colon, ensuring a harmonized filter to let out precisely what needs to be expelled and keep in that which needs to be reabsorbed. Your ability to achieve this balance with your larger life circumstances is also improved as the orange color infuses your root and sacral chakras. Every drop of the orange liquid is used by your body.

The liquid in the second vial is transparent and yellow. It is full of the electrolytes your body needs to bring your minerals back into balance after having diarrhea episodes. Drink in the yellow liquid, which is full of potassium, magnesium, calcium, and a variety of other mineral compounds. Watch and feel these substances moving into your cells to help them regain energy.

Finally, take your hands, rub them together to create an accumulation of energy, and place them on your gut. Breathe in the healing life-force energy to this part of your body, asking your body's inherent healing capacity to restore your gut to even better functioning than before you had diarrhea. When you have completed this exercise, release your hands and return to the present moment.

Meditation: Engage in an emptiness meditation by sitting with and savoring the inner part of you that feels still and empty—the part of you open to the vastness of existence. Explore the void within and see what you discover. Write your findings in a journal.

Ear Infection (Otitis Media)

Physical description: A bacterial or viral infection in the inner ear, causing inflammation and swelling and potentially resulting in discharge, pain, and temporary loss of hearing.

Energy center(s): Root, throat

Nourishment: *Diet*—(1) Reduce or eliminate simple sugars, such as white sugar, honey, fruit juice, and baked goods, as they tend to impair immune function; (2) Aim to eat a healthy diet full of whole foods that are high in nutrient density to ensure an intake of vitamins and minerals that are essential in supporting the immune system (e.g., zinc, vitamin C). *Supplements*—(1) A high-quality multivitamin containing vitamin A, vitamin C, and zinc; (2) Xylitol in the form of chewing gum, lozenges, or liquids has shown to be effective in reducing the occurrence of ear infections; (3) Zinc lozenges for short-term use during an infectious episode; (4) Extra vitamin C taken throughout the day to support immune function.

Emotion(s): Anger at something that has been heard, feeling inauthentic

Limiting belief(s): I refuse to listen. I am furious with and pained by what I heard. I tune people out. Doesn't anyone listen to me?

Power animal: Wolf

Flower essence(s): Scarlet Monkeyflower, Star Tulip, Trumpet Vine

Affirmation(s): I am open to my inner and outer voice. My ears help me to pay attention to what I need to hear. I respond to what I hear in an authentic way for me.

Visualization: Tune into the location of your ears. Tilt your head to the right as you expose your left ear. In your mind's eye, construct a funnel shape and direct the point of the funnel towards the opening in your ear. This special two-way funnel allows for the release and replacement of any notions, beliefs, thoughts, or things you have heard with your ear. Imagine the funnel circulates a shaft of warm, healing, bluish light into the spiraled structure of the inner ear.

As the light unwinds its coiled structure, it clears out anything clogging the ear. See outdated or negatively charged words, images, beliefs, and ideas, and allow them to be attracted and cling to the corkscrew of light penetrating the deep recesses of your ear. Let them attach to the light like ornaments. Perhaps you notice some debris, excessive wax, or microorganisms that you'd like to expel; let these cling to the light. Each time the shaft of light picks up an object, it turns a deeper blue. Once you feel your eardrum has been properly cleared, remove the funnel structure and discard it.

Now imagine creating, in the palm of your hand, a pyramidal structure embedded with ancient Egyptian healing energy. Place the point of the pyramid into the entrance to the eardrum and allow the healing words, symbols, chants, and prayers to unravel into your ear and coat it completely and fully. Your left ear is now laced with ancient divinity and will allow you to receive only what is in alignment with your true purpose and sacred path.

Bring your head to center, take a deep breath, and see the breath traveling not only to the depths of your belly, but also to your ears. When you exhale, see all you need to release being expelled through the breath and out your ears.

Now repeat the same exercise with the right ear.

Meditation: Find a sound that is nourishing for you—whether that be the sound(s) heard by holding your ear to a conch shell, by being in nature and passively taking in the sounds, or even by using a small musical instrument to play a couple of notes that are pacifying to you. During the meditation, focus only on the sounds. See the sounds you are listening to travel into your ears to carry out any stuck auditory debris.

Eczema (Atopic Dermatitis)

Physical description: A skin disorder characterized by inflamed, itchy, scaly lesions.

Energy center(s): Root

Nourishment: *Diet*—(1) Work with a qualified health professional to identify food allergies; (2) As much as possible, avoid inflammatory foods, such as those that are highly processed (those high in sugar and/or trans fat) or contain dairy, gluten, alcohol, and animal products; (3) Eat wild-caught salmon or, if vegetarian, incorporate flaxseed oil into your daily regimen. *Supplements*—(1) Multivitamin containing essential nutrients for healthy skin: vitamin A, the B complex, vitamin C, vitamin D, and vitamin E, along with zinc; (2) Omega-3 fatty acids in the form of fish or flaxseed oil; (3) Botanicals reducing allergy responses, such as quercetin, green-tea extract, and licorice.

Emotion(s): Irritation (especially about the environment)

Limiting belief(s): I am irritated by someone or something in my environment; this person or thing gets under my skin. My identity is threatened. I am unable to trust my surroundings. My situation is old and crusty.

Power animal: Fish

Flower essence(s): Dill

Affirmation(s): I trust my surroundings and know they support me. I am in the right place in the right moment. I am fluid and flexible in the coolness of my skin. When the time is right, I ease out of situations with grace and ease.

Visualization: Visualize the expanse of your skin as a landscape. With your mind's eye, travel over the valleys and hills, the flatlands, the moist and dry parts, the forested areas. What has this landscape witnessed? What stories does it need to tell? Sit in silence, allowing your skin to speak.

Now travel to the places on your body where you have eczema. See these sites as areas on the landscape where battles have occurred. What was being fought? What continues to make you irritated, inflamed, and crusty? Zoom in closer to see what the inflammation, the fire, is about. Let your skin speak to you about what it is fighting against to protect you.

Take a deep breath in, and, with the coolness of the air you take in, release these patches of fire from your burning skin. Allow your breath to move to each part of your inflamed skin, putting out any fires, itching, oozing, or tenderness.

See the collective wounds and inflammation travel like lava out your limbs—through your fingers and toes—making their way to the moist, cool earth. The earth generously transforms this inflamed, fiery energy into a cooling, healing salve. You welcome the healing offered by the earth. The salve begins to permeate your limbs and spread over the landscape of your skin, coating it with a layer of trust and protection. Your battle scars begin to radiate with the peace of surrender to what is best for you. You feel calm and soothed. You and the environment are one.

Meditation: Meditate on your relationship with your everyday environment. Make a list of all the things (people, events, situations) that make you irritated. Now make another list of ways you can empower and trust yourself to overcome or solve these irritations.

Emotional Eating

Physical description: Responding to emotional events by eating food rather than expressing the emotion felt.

Energy center(s): Sacral, throat

Nourishment: There are three steps to shifting from emotional eating to purposeful eating: (1) *Become aware.* Practice being in touch with your body and emotions by cultivating the distinction between when you are physically hungry (physical hunger builds over time and does not demand specific foods typically high in salt, fat, and/or sugar) versus when you need to emotionally express (i.e., after an emotional event); (2) *Implement alternatives.* If you feel vulnerable to emotional eating, find something you can do instead of eating, like journaling, calling a friend, or taking a brief, fifteen-minute walk; (3) *Get to the root.* Understand why you are engaging with emotional eating. What is the emotion that needs to be expressed? Find healthy, safe ways you can express these emotions before they pile up as food!

Emotion(s): Feeling unfulfilled, shame, fear of one's feelings or their expression, guilt, any emotions not expressed (anger, fear, grief, etc.)

Limiting belief(s): I control my emotions by stuffing them down with food. Eating is the only thing that comforts me. I am a terrible person for feeling this way.

Power animal: Otter

Flower essence(s): Cerato, Chaparral, Fuchsia

Affirmation(s): I release all that needs to surface in a healthy, positive way. I am fulfilled by my life experiences. I flow with people, places, and events in a fluid manner.

Visualization: Place your hands, one on top of another, on your low belly. Breathe deeply so your hands rise up on the inhale and release on the exhale.

Using your gift of inner vision, look deep into your abdomen area to see whether you have any stored anger, fear, or guilt lodged inside, wanting to be set free. Call forth any and all of these emotions, allowing them to pinwheel through you, spinning and spinning with increasing momentum in the core of your being, until, finally, the emotion(s) spin(s) out of your body.

Now that you have extra space within you, where the emotions have vacated, fill in the space with the energy of movement and creativity. Allow your wizard self to sparkle, waving a wand and showering stars of potential in front of you, on your path forward.

Breathe in to prepare yourself for another release of emotion. And this time, feel in your belly region any sadness, loneliness, and grief that have lodged themselves within you like heavy rocks. Maybe you even feel them weighing down your chest. With the help of your deep breath, imagine they are thrown far away and hit the ground, shattering to pieces. Each piece dissolves into the earth and, in the process, becomes transformed into seeds. You watch these seeds begin to sprout and flower before you, as if in accelerated time. Your sadness, grief, and loneliness have become peace and beauty. With your inner eyes, you take in the flowers' beautiful colors, and you can smell their intense fragrance wafting through the air on the light breeze.

With your hands still cupped on your belly, grounded with the anchor of your breath, dive deep into the ocean of your bowels. Put all awareness into the watery depths of your emotional body. Feel your body's ability to become fluid and flowing, washing through any stuck fear from past, present, or future. In this moment, your body becomes timeless and vast. You feel whole and complete without having the heavy burden of fear limiting your actions, specifically your eating. A gush of fresh, clean water makes its way through the tunnel of your intestines, clearing away any emotional sludge, expelling it through your feet. Your belly feels soft and clean.

Imagine a waterwheel or pinwheel placed in this area of your body. See any anger, grief, or fear, as well as any other stuck emotions, put into motion on this wheel, being dispersed from your being in a healthy way instead of getting stuck within you, causing you to eat for emotional reasons.

In this perfect moment and in all perfect moments to come, your body knows physical hunger sensations, and you act on your physical hunger cues, honoring your body's inherent wisdom. Any emotional eating attempts or inclinations are thrown off, like the water tossed from the wheel, moving through your body. You are in absolute harmony with your body's rhythm to eat.

Meditation: What is your favorite food to eat when you are eating emotionally? Reflect on the food; see it as a symbol or a metaphor for what you are really experiencing. Note how it is connected to your thought patterns and your childhood, and meditate on what you could choose instead of the food next time you are feeling like engaging in emotional eating.

Enlarged Prostate (See Prostate Problems)

Esophageal Reflux (See Heartburn)

Excessive Appetite

Physical description: A propensity to ingest more food (calories) than is needed for energy expenditure.

Energy center(s): Root, sacral, solar plexus, throat, third eye

Nourishment: *Diet*—(1) Observe and track your hunger before and after a meal by using a simple rating scale (one equals very hungry, ravenous; ten equals painfully full). See if you can keep your intake to a level of about five (no hunger) rather than to feelings of uncomfortable fullness; (2) Balance blood sugar by eating foods low on the glycemic index (e.g., nonstarchy vegetables, legumes, lean protein, whole grains) and by avoiding simple sugars; (3) Eat small, frequent meals throughout the day to help keep blood sugar levels stable. *Supplements*—(1) High-quality multivitamin to ensure all vitamin and mineral needs are being met; (2) Digestive-enzyme supplement taken with the meal so foods eaten and digested and assimilated rather than excreted.

Emotion(s): Longing, loneliness, grief for lack of passion and purpose

Limiting belief(s): I feel empty. I long for fulfillment. It's never enough. My life is a bottomless pit. I've lost my sense of instinct.

Power animal: Squirrel

Flower essence(s): Angelica, California Pitcher Plant, California Wild Rose

Affirmation(s): I am nourished by life. I am utterly fulfilled by living. Instinct and intuition guide my life's path.

Visualization: Close your eyes and take a deep breath to center your-self fully in the moment.

Imagine you find yourself on a sunny island full of fruit trees. The sun is radiant and warm, and you take in its dazzling rays through your skin. Each photon of light from the sun carries with it the joy of living, and the longer you bask in its glow, the more every cell in your body becomes infused with the presence of the sun. Slowly and steadily, every cell drinks in the sunlight and feels invigorated.

You notice all of your cells, starting with those of the head and working your way down to those of your feet, have become like tiny individual suns, each of them glowing with the potential of your being. All negativity, stuck emotions, resentment from the past, unre-solved anger dissolves in the presence of the magnificent power and presence of the sunlight. You feel empowered and inspired. The rib-bon of your life's path, which you see before you, feels complete and dynamic, and at once, you feel confident you can conquer all of life's challenges.

You receive information that the fruit growing in this field is of a different nature than fruit in the usual, physical realm. Each tree car-ries with it an essence or quality imparted in the fruit. Eating these fruits would help you to become fulfilled on the inside in deep ways. Often times, we try to find satisfaction and fulfillment in eating. In this eating experience, you are released from that bond or tie to insa-tiable eating.

You come upon two trees that seem to have significant value to you. One is a tree bearing a bright orange, juicy fruit you have never tasted before. As you bite into it, you receive a burst of joy that travels through your body. With each successive bite, you come to the real-ization that you would like to invite more passion, pleasure, and play into your life, specifically into your relationships with others. This fruit helps you to uncover the beauty of your childlike self, who has spent so much time hiding within you. You invite your child self to make an appearance when you are eating food and when you are out having fun with friends. With the last bite of this brilliantly orange fruit, you can see the beauty of the potential of your creativity blos-soming by being open to the mystery of being playful and fun.

Your body feels relaxed, and a smile expands on your face. Life is joyous and full of pleasure and dance. You open your arms to the sky, absorbing even more of the sun essence, drinking in the rays, and becoming energized with the magic of life.

With your next breath, you skip forward to the next tree, which is a wispy, yet durable tree bearing a bright yellow-orange fruit—similar to the color of a sunset. You have never seen this fruit before, but you are intrigued by its soft, inviting texture. Taking a generous bite, you realize this fruit imparts the message of sweetness in a way that goes beyond what sugar provides.

You begin to reflect on all the aspects of your life that do not feel sweet to you anymore. They have become mundane, lackluster, and even demanding. Any feelings of deprivation within you come to the surface of your being. You look at them more closely, asking yourself, "Where do I feel deprived and depleted?" As you continue to take bites from this gorgeous fruit, you see these situations in your life transform to benefit your highest good. You see the steps you need to take to make these transformations. They do not feel overwhelming, but well within your realm of control. You give gratitude to the fruit and the tree for this insight. You have sealed up this information within so you can act on it in the perfect moment.

You take a seat on the warm island sand, looking ahead to the horizon before you, and the expanse of the blue-green ocean fills your awareness. With a gentle breath carried in from the playful breeze, you breathe in and savor all the messages you have received from the two trees of wisdom on this mystical island—those of pleasure, play, passion, and true sweetness. Your being has been transformed, and you have let go any need to overeat or excessively eat. You have replaced that need with qualities that are much more fulfilling than any food could ever offer. Cultivate these fruits within you with daily practice and appreciation, and you will always feel nourished.

Meditation: Reflect on what you could do abundantly that would be nourishing, good, and healthy for your being (e.g., giving others hugs, volunteering an extra hour for a noteworthy cause you have passion for, spending extra time in a relaxing bath).

Farsightedness

Physical description: Difficulty seeing near objects clearly.

Energy center(s): Third eye

Nourishment: *Diet*—(1) Eat foods high in the yellow plant pigment lutein, such as green, leafy vegetables (e.g., spinach); (2) Include dietary sources of omega-3 fats, such as fish, leafy greens, nuts, and seeds (e.g., flaxseed meal/oil). *Supplements*—A high-quality multivitamin containing vitamins A, C, and E, and zinc.

Emotion(s): Fear of the obvious

Limiting belief(s): I neglect my own needs. I refuse to see the obvious. I ignore messages, signs, and visions presented to me in the present moment. I cannot focus.

Power animal: Eagle

Flower essence(s): Blackberry, Penstemon, Queen Anne's Lace

Affirmation(s): I see with clarity what is front of me. My inner vision is aligned with my outer sight. I notice "insight-full" details.

Visualization: Close your eyes. Relax them behind the padding of your soft eyelids.

Using the vision of your third eye, cast forth a beam of light in front of you, almost as if you were wearing a headlamp. And with this dazzling beam of light, create a small indigo sphere about the size of a softball. Make it translucent, but with substance. It is soft and malleable, but strong and durable, like an eyeball. Let this shape provide you with a reflection of your own internal vision. The images are trapped within the territory of your third eye.

Hold this sphere comfortably, within both hands, in front of you, as if it were a crystal ball. Imagine for a moment that this sphere represents the essence of your vision, of the external and internal worlds you are exposed to and that you create. Sit back and relax, and allow all the images within your field of sight to float through the beautiful orb you hold. Observe images, scenes, and scenarios, as if you were watching a movie. Do any of them speak to you more than others? Which ones seem to be sticky and represent unresolved issues that need some further scrutiny?

Choose an image and let it move out from the sphere and into the free space in front of you to enable it to animate. Let it come alive. Allow it to get close and personal. With your perfect vision, examine it from all angles. Magnify it as much as possible to see what is really at work here. Do you feel any discomfort with its proximity?

What are your body sensations telling you? Watch it transform until it becomes so detailed that it appears pixilated, composed of many tiny dots of color, like a pointillist painting. Does your attachment to the image change? What colors make up the image? What is your feeling about the animation? How does it feel to be so close? What do you see that you perhaps did not recognize before? What can you add to the image or situation that was not there before, but improves or benefits it? Take a deep breath, if you need to draw upon your intuition for answers, and wait patiently for responses.

When you are ready, zoom out of the animation so you are back to visioning the indigo orb once again. Hold it carefully with an intention of clarity and focus. Stream a beam of bright indigo light from your forehead into this sphere. See the light dancing within it, especially as you move it within your hands. Close your hands around the sphere and watch it shrink until it becomes the size of a marble. Raise the small marble to your forehead. In a second, your forehead drinks in the indigo energy of light from the marble and sends it down to both your eyes, rejuvenating and invigorating them with the energy of clarity and the ability to take a careful look at situations to see where there might be lessons and hidden messages. With this amazing focusing ability, your eyes can now see objects that are close to you with utter clarity.

Rub your hands together until they become slightly warm and then cup them over your eyes. Open your eyes to the darkness they are veiled in. Mentally affirm, "My inner vision provides me with clarity and focus." When you have absorbed the energy that you created in your palms, let your hands fall away and your eyes open to the miracle of life and rainbow of possibilities that surround you.

Meditation: Fix your gaze on one point close to your eyes, where you might normally have difficulty seeing. Meditate on this point until it becomes more focused, and then close your eyes and start again. Repeat for a couple of minutes every day.

Fatigue

Physical description: Fatigue is a general sense of exhaustion and depleted energy reserves that may be an indicator of excessive stress, insufficient and lack of good-quality sleep, overwork, and/or poor nutrition. Although fatigue may result in response to a single event, its repeated occurrence may denote the presence of chronic underlying health conditions, such as bacterial or viral infections, toxicity, food allergies, impaired immune status, or low thyroid function, to name a few.

Energy center(s): Root, solar plexus, third eye

Nourishment: *Diet*—(1) Eat foods that are energy promoting rather than energy draining—whole foods, like fruits, vegetables, whole grains and beans, rather than processed food products depleted of a complex array of plant compounds; (2) Avoid high-sugar foods and eat foods ranking low on the glycemic index; (3) Eat small, frequent meals throughout the day to keep your energy balanced; (4) Minimize or exclude caffeinated beverages, as they tend to mask fatigue; (5) Work with a qualified healthcare professional to identify food allergies; (6) If you are anemic, eat iron-rich foods (see entry for "Anemia"). *Supplements*—A high-quality multivitamin that contains the entire B complex, plus vitamin C.

Emotion(s): Unworthiness, shame, fear

Limiting belief(s): I am filled with emptiness. I cannot overcome all that is presented to me. I am a void. I am tired of living and lack energy for all of life's challenges.

Power animal: Salmon

Flower essence(s): Morning Glory, Oak, Peppermint

Affirmation(s): Life presents me with opportunities. I am saturated with the energy needed to be satisfied with living. I weave passion into all I do. Purpose fills me.

Visualization: Imagine you are walking in a green grassy field full of a variety of trees. The air feels fresh and light. You breathe in deeply, letting the summer air infuse your body from head to toe. And with this breath, you become the essence of summer: ripe, sweet, full of potential and brilliance.

The green grass and soil underneath your bare feet feels cool and soothing and connects you to the energy of the earth. You can see the bottoms of your feet sprout roots, like a plant. With each breath you take, those roots become thicker and stronger, and they find their way deeper into the loamy soil and clay layers of the earth. You feel strengthened by your connection with the earth in this way. Through those roots, you become nourished with the earth's healing energy, which travels up from the molten core of the earth into the tips of your roots. It continues up to your feet, courses through the stretch of your legs and then finally plants itself into the base of your spine. This energy feels electric within you, running a current of enthusiasm all along your being. You realize how good it feels to be alive.

You extend your arms overhead, reaching towards the pale blue sky, and in a moment, your arms become branches of a tree. By looking down at the rest of your body, you notice you have transformed into a unique, large tree. Your arms never get tired as they are supported by the life energy coming into you from the earth, and they gently sway in the comfort of the warm summer air. They are so nourished by life force that they become populated with more branches and a multitude of shiny, thick green leaves. Each leaf sings with joy as it extends its face towards the warm sun, absorbing its healing light so it can photosynthesize and grow with opportunities. Tiny birds come to rest in your branchlike arms. They create their own song in unison.

You are fed completely by this experience. The love you generate forms blossoms of potential, passion, and purpose on your branches. With your repeating breaths, the blossoms grow into succulent, ripe fruits of all types. They are full of juicy sweetness. You feel complete and fulfilled as this bountiful tree, soaking in energy from the soil and filtering in the light of the universe. You are fed by your fruits and by what you have to offer to all those you meet.

And, in an instant, with the movement of your breath, your arms whisk down to be by your sides. All of the fruits, blossoms, leaves, birds, and branches are now a part of who you are. You pick up each foot, one at a time, and feel the invisible earthy energy grounding you, making you fully present in this moment. You feel the aliveness of your spirit. Every cell in your being is bathed in possibilities.

Meditation: Make a list of everything you are currently *doing*, and then compare that to a list of what you are currently *being*. See how the two lists match up.

Fatty Liver (SEE LIVER PROBLEMS)

Fever

Physical description: An increase in the body's internal temperature, suggesting the presence of infection or disease.

Energy center(s): Root

Nourishment: *Diet*—Focus intake primarily on liquids (broths, distilled water, juices).

Emotion(s): Anger, irritation, feeling overwhelmed

Limiting belief(s): My anger takes me over. I am being invaded. I am boiling inside.

Power animal: Dolphin

Flower essence(s): Aloe Vera

Affirmation(s): I let my emotions flow through me in a cool and calm manner. I see the divine intention in all events. I remain calm, cool, and collected.

Visualization: If you have a fever, envision it manifesting in your body as if you have taken on the form of a house on fire. Look at the house from a distance rather than being in the midst of the flames. Scan your body, as if you were a firefighter surveying a scene where he or she is about to intervene.

Rather than view the fire as a nuisance or an emergency, communicate with it to understand what it is trying to say. Dialogue with the flames as though they were people, or facets of yourself, with messages. What do they say? Try to listen as best you can. Quiet your inner self, observe the brilliant light of the flames, now separate from the house, and put your gaze in the center of the flames. Lose yourself deeper and deeper within the dance and rhythm of this bundle of fire that obviously has something to express. Your breath feeds the flames and allows them to dance and communicate as they wish.

Pause here for a couple of moments to get feedback.

The more you permit the fire to roar and burn, the more it begins to slowly subside. Little by little, it begins to lose its momentum. Whatever needed purifying and cleansing has received it in perfect amounts.

Continue to stare into the flames. Note whether any images appear to you. If so, apply their significance to your life situation.

Does anything about these images need clearing or to be dissolved? If your answer is yes, let the images melt into the body of the flame, which is now becoming cool white rather than a blazing hot orange-red. If there are any other aspects of your life that do not serve your life's path, the white flame before you is willing to transform it into that which is good, true, and beautiful for your inner self. Take a couple of moments to reflect on that which you feel ready to let go of for good and pure reasons. When you are ready, toss them into the white, brilliant flame of inspiration and transformation.

Collectively, all of these items, events, and images coalesce to become a phoenix—a powerful bird that opens its expanse of wing to embrace you. You walk into the embrace of the phoenix, and you are surrounded with blinding white light. This light permeates every cell of your body, cooling it down from any fever and invigorating your immune system to bring you back into balance. With each breath you take, the phoenix expands and closes her wings around you in a very motherlike, nurturing manner. You feel at peace—calm, cool, and collected.

And then you begin to realize that you are the phoenix. The white light slowly begins to pixelate around you and eventually becomes completely swallowed up in your being. Your eyes are open, and you examine your body, noticing a glow of purity enveloping you. Your immune system feels strong, and any fever symptoms are letting go, to be replaced with perfect health and vitality.

Meditation: Use the image of fire as one that represents purification and clarification. Meditate on the flames while you envision sending stored packages of emotions into a fiery dance to be purified and clarified, so their true purpose in your life may be revealed.

Fibromyalgia

Physical description: A generalized disorder consisting of chronic muscle and tissue pain at designated points on the body.

Energy center(s): Root, third eye

Nourishment: *Diet*—(1) Work with a qualified healthcare professional to identify food allergies; (2) Limit or avoid sugar, alcohol, and caffeine; (3) Eat organically grown, unprocessed foods as much as possible—fresh fruits and vegetables, whole grains, and legumes. *Supplements*—(1) A high-quality, high-potency multivitamin and mineral; (2) Additional magnesium to assist in the production of cellular energy and to reduce pain and tenderness; (3) 5-hydroxytryptophan (5-HTP) to lesson pain and stiffness and improve sleep quality.

Emotion(s): Grief, anger at being neglected, fear of being abandoned

Limiting belief(s): I have shut down my instincts and intuition. Living is painful. My pain provides distraction from doing what I need to for myself. I am burdened.

Power animal: Antelope

Flower essence(s): Centaury, Clematis, Dogwood, Mugwort, Peppermint, Quince

Affirmation(s): I nurture my whole self, using the information I receive from my instincts and intuition. I am free and full of light and love for life. I move gracefully to the flow of life.

Visualization: *Shake your body out very lightly before doing this exercise. Engage and encourage the flow of life force throughout your body. Do this movement only to the level of comfort. When you are ready to begin the visualization, it is best if you can lie down, preferably on something soft, like a bed.*

Close your eyes, have your arms and hands at your sides, and imagine you are lying within an enclosed structure that resembles a tanning bed. The top shield encloses the front of your body, and there is a sliver of an opening on both right and left sides. It is roomy enough on the inside to give you a comfortable sensation. You feel warm and safe within this enclosure, and as you sink into it and relax, its shape becomes more organic and molds to the soft shape of your body.

It now takes on the appearance of the familiar shape of an oyster shell. It is made from natural materials, opalescent and slightly reflective on the inside and textured on the outside. Being enrobed in its structure imparts a feeling of security; it brings forth a connection with being alive and even a safe feeling of being within a womb.

After a couple of seconds, you begin to hear the rush of the ocean waves, almost as if your ear were fastened to a conch shell. The heavenly sound ripples through your whole being, cascading from top to bottom. Eventually, the flow of your body moves in concert with the constant peace and consistency of the echoing of the ocean waves. Old feelings and any bodily pain are cast away to the waves moving through your body, and they are replaced by generous infusions of nourishment of body, heart, and soul. The pull of the ocean current takes this nourishment into the places that need it most, and wherever it lands, it swirls like an eddy, filling the space completely.

At once, a feeling of lightness washes through your being. Any tenderness, pain, heaviness dissolves in the roar of the ocean waves. Soon you realize that you have expanded your consciousness beyond the limitations of your body. You have become the ocean. The boundaries of your body have evaporated and been replaced with the qualities of the ocean—its vastness and depth. You recognize your ability to be limitless and infinite. The salt of the ocean that you feel within your essence reminds you of your connection with the earth, with the earth's mineralized groundedness. The ocean and the earth are one, swirling together like yin and yang. You are the green and the blue, the marble of the planet, and at the same time, you are the galaxy of stars, the universe—nothingness and everything all at once.

Now bring your awareness back to the outline of your body. Acknowledge your beautiful form, the alchemy of water and earth coming together within you. Feel healing rays of blue and green light streaming through your body, providing nurturing, healing, and wisdom from a deep place. When the time feels right, and you've absorbed enough of the glow of health, come back to your place in the shell structure, letting it morph back into a rectangular tanning bed and then disappearing, leaving you on your own bed, safe and sound.

In your own time, sit up slowly, open your eyes, sway your body back and forth to remember the ocean waves moving within you, and say aloud, "I move gracefully to the flow of life."

Meditation: Place your palms about two inches apart or to the level at which you feel a gentle, magnetic tension between your hands. Feel this energy as a small symbol of the great, powerful energy that invigorates you. Meditate on this feeling and see if you can strengthen it with your intention to do so.

Once you feel the energy flowing in your hands, place them on parts of your body that feel sore, stiff, or painful. See the ribbons of energy coursing from your hands into these areas, relieving them of their burden and pain, and infusing them with renewed energy.

Flu (See Viral Infection)

Foot Pain (Bunions, Hammertoes)

Physical description: A bunion occurs when the big toe tilts in towards the second toe, causing the inner foot to take on an angled appearance. Hammertoes are muscular deformities in the toes, which result in them appearing bent. Both can lead to structural and even functional changes of the foot.

Energy center(s): Root

Nourishment: *Diet*—Eat cooling, anti-inflammatory foods such as raw vegetables (especially leafy greens), fish (high in anti-inflammatory fats), whole grains, nuts, and seeds, while minimizing or avoiding red meat. *Supplements*—(1) A high-quality multivitamin and mineral containing vitamin D, calcium, and magnesium; (2) Omega-3 fatty-acid supplement (from fish or flaxseed oils) to help reduce inflammation; (3) Botanical anti-inflammatories, such as ginger, quercetin, curcumin, and boswellia.

Emotion(s): Insecurity, distraction, disconnection

Limiting belief(s): I cannot stand up for myself. My connection to the physical world is altered in such a way that causes me pain. I neglect my ability to ground to the earth. I refuse to rely on others for support.

Power animal: Goat

Flower essence(s): California Poppy, Corn, Larkspur

Affirmation(s): I stand tall and firmly planted. My stance is strong and stable. I accept my existence as a human being. I am sure-footed and welcome support from others.

Visualization: Find yourself seated on a deserted beach at sunset. The sun is slowing dropping into the horizon. The sand beneath your bare feet is warm from the heat of the sun during the day. You stand up and gently push your feet, one by one, into the tiny quartz crystal sand, allowing them to be covered completely.

Every tiny granule of sand pulses its infinite energy into the bottom of your feet, relieving all blocks and hardened tissue. Your soles feel soft and supple. They begin to pulse with the rhythm of the fine quartz, stimulating all the acupressure points in the feet, which go to all the organs in the body, and invigorating them with this subtle vibration. The sand crystals covering the top and sides of your feet begin pulsing this energy through to the toes. Any stagnant energy or pain is broken up by the constant pulsations, sending all that needs releasing through the tips of the toes, like a stream of energy.

You feel a cool, electric energy radiating through your feet, opening them up to the feeling of being connected with the earth. This cool energy has dissipated all heat, swelling, and redness.

You remove your feet from the sand and begin to walk on the beach with your feet feeling free and light. The white, cooling, electric energy of the sand crystals radiates through every toe. With every step, you feel more invigorated and alive. You become aware of all of your surroundings, and the intensity of the sunset washes over you. You thank your feet for carrying you everywhere you choose to go and for being the messengers that bring in the energy of the earth to nourish your whole self!

Meditation: Take five minutes to massage your feet, or have someone else massage them while you relax in silence.

Gallstones

Physical description: The accumulation of bile products, ranging from cholesterol to bile salts, which collect and crystallize in the gallbladder, potentially obstructing the flow of bile and resulting in inflammation.

Energy center(s): Solar plexus

Nourishment: *Diet*—(1) Eat a low-fat, high-fiber diet composed of whole, unprocessed (plant) foods like vegetables (nonstarchy), whole grains, legumes, seeds, and nuts; (2) Avoid foods that are high in sugar or those that have been fried; (3) Reduce saturated (animal) fat and substitute with unsaturated fats (e.g., seed oils, olive oil); (4) If you have gallstones, avoid caffeine, as it stimulates gallbladder contractions; (5) Drink adequate water; (6) Work with a qualified healthcare professional to identify food allergies. *Supplements*—(1) Soluble fiber supplement (e.g., pectin, guar gum, psyllium); (2) A high-quality, multivitamin and mineral that contains vitamins C and E; (3) Phosphatidylcholine (lecithin) to improve cholesterol solubility in bile; (4)

Botanicals to facilitate bile secretion, such as artichoke, milk thistle, dandelion, turmeric.

Emotion(s): Fury, rage, indecision, helplessness

Limiting belief(s): I have become hardened with hate. I resent my past.

Power animal: Monkey

Flower essence(s): Dogwood, Golden Ear Drops, Larch, Star of Bethlehem

Affirmation(s): All bitterness in my life has dissolved. I embrace the integration of opposites in my life. My past flows into the present in a harmonious rhythm.

Visualization: Close your eyes and focus on your emotional body. From your emotional body, extend armlike projections or emotional feelers to locate places where resentment and bitterness have taken up residence in your body. Where have these feelings collected? Look for places in the body that have become rigid or calcified—indica tions of collected feelings.

If you have gallstones, zoom in to your gallbladder and look closely. Let your emotional feelers wrap around it to sense the events or people that resentment or hardness have been directed towards. With this information, direct loving kindness towards whatever you have accumulated bitterness about, and mentally affirm, "I bless and release you from my life."

Untangle your emotional feeler from the gallbladder, and with the brilliant insight of your mind's eye, nestled in your forehead, transform the gallstones into quartz crystals. Your gallbladder is now holding a sac of tiny quartz crystals; quartz is very healing and nourishing for your overall energy field and assists in bringing you into a state of balance. Next, use the laserlike properties of your third eye to break up the quartz crystals into fine powder. Take a generous deep breath in, and with a strong exhale, blow the powder so a fine puff of quartz blankets your whole being. By doing so, you impart the qualities of balance and justice to the essence of your being. Do this a couple more times if you feel you need additional work on this aspect.

When you are finished, your gallbladder will be clear and fully functioning. Its activity is now harmonized with that of its partner, the liver, and the quartz powder in your energy field soaks through to your heart and circulation to help regulate your body's production of cholesterol and other fats. Feel the physical extension and emotional release in your abdomen, and feel invigoration coursing throughout your body. Going forward, any time you feel judgmental or bitter, enrobe yourself in this fine quartz powder.

When you feel comfortable with your visualization results, return your emotional body back to your physical body, and become aware and fully present.

Meditation: Engage in a laughing meditation in which you recall an event in your life that made you chuckle. Begin to laugh and let it amplify, vibrating your belly. Relax into the laughter and feel the effects in your upper abdomen. Now think of something that makes you angry and, instead of becoming mad, make yourself laugh about it.

Genital Warts (SEE VENEREAL DISEASE)

Gonorrhea (SEE VENEREAL DISEASE)

Gout

Physical description: Accumulation of uric acid (a product of the metabolism of one of the units of DNA and RNA called purines) in the bloodstream and deposition of uric acid–containing crystals in joints, tendons, and tissues.

Energy center(s): Root

Nourishment: *Diet*—(1) Avoid dietary triggers like alcohol, organ meats, simple sugars (white sugar, honey, corn syrup), and excessive protein. (In general, aim for the recommended daily allowance of 0.8 grams of protein per kilogram of body weight, unless you are pregnant or lactating. A 70 kg [154 lb] person would need about 56 grams of protein per day.) (2) Consume a high-fiber, low-fat diet consisting primarily of plant-based foods, like whole grains, vegetables, nuts, and seeds; (3) Drink copious amount of water to promote the excretion of uric acid. *Supplements*—(1) Anti-inflammatories such as omega-3 fatty acids (from fish or flaxseed oils), bromelain, and quercetin; (2) Folic acid (a B vitamin) to reduce the formation of uric acid by the body; (3) A high-potency multivitamin and mineral.

Emotion(s): Feeling inflamed and infuriated by an inability to move forward; insecurity; rage towards family

Limiting belief(s): My anger pains me. When I am "in-raged," I feel caged. There are too many challenges to moving forward. I can't run fast enough from my past into my future.

Power animal: Panther

Flower essence(s): Aloe Vera, Impatiens, Sage, Trillium, Willow

Affirmation(s): I move with grace and ease. I accept my origins. Anger propels me to action if I choose.

Visualization: In your hands, you hold a laser device that is a small wand about six inches long. With the power and focus of your intention, you are able to turn on and direct the laser to dissolve crystals of uric acid that have lodged within your joints, especially your feet.

Take a deep breath and tune in to the areas of your body that have collected uric acid in excessive amounts, causing you pain. With your mind, turn on the red laser beam, which is about one-quarter inch in diameter, and move it to where you feel pain from the crystals. Once you have found a place, shatter the uric-acid crystals with the laser beam. Allow them to be pulverized to a fine mist and then evaporate from the confines of your body. Repeat the process until you feel that you have cleared your body of unhealthy pools of uric acid.

When you have completed this procedure, imagine you are standing on a slab of pure quartz crystal. The quartz acts as an energetic magnet to remove all metabolic debris from your cells. You watch, with your inner vision, how substances start to move out of cells and stream down through your body, out of your feet and into the crystal. Several rivulets of substances, all in parallel with your energy meridians, trace through your body vertically, from head to toe, to be deposited into the quartz reservoir. After a couple of seconds for this streaming to occur, scan your body and notice how clear it is. All stagnation, sluggishness, and stubbornness have been removed.

Let light from the quartz beneath you radiate upwards through your feet and into the pillars of your legs and the rest of your body, infusing you with the ability to become and embrace your ability to be open to change and love. The organs in your body responsible for the excretion of uric acid, mainly your kidneys and gut, are saturated with this light and are filled with the ease of being able to let go of painful events, situations, or anything that holds you back from your potential and passion.

The light of the quartz begins to dissipate, and the quartz slowly disappears from under your feet, traveling back into the inner realm of the earth. The laser in your hand goes into your toolkit for whenever you may need it to break up any stuck energy in your body.

Meditation: Place a small quartz crystal on the areas of your body that you feel are gouty. Meditate on the transfer of uric-acid crystals to the quartz crystal. Allow the quartz to absorb your pain.

Grief

Physical description: An overwhelming feeling of loss that can result in a sad or depressed disposition.

Energy center(s): Sacral, heart, third eye, crown

Nourishment: *Diet*—(1) Eat green vegetables (e.g., broccoli, spinach) to open up the heart chakra; (2) Focus on food sources of omega-3 fatty acids, such as fish, flaxseed meal/oil, nuts, seeds, and leafy green vegetables to ensure adequate healthy fats for the brain. *Supplements*—A fish or flaxseed oil supplement to supply omega-3 fats.

Emotion(s): Grief spans the emotional spectrum from numbness and being distant to despair and anxiety to sadness and loneliness.

Limiting belief(s): I am alone and abandoned. No one can understand the loss I endure. My heart cannot handle this tragedy.

Power animal: Bear

Flower essence(s): Bleeding Heart, Chaparral, Mustard, Scotch Broom

Affirmation(s): My heart blossoms with growth and gratitude for every aspect of my life. Within the seeming imperfection lies the ultimate divine perfection. I embrace the unknown with compassion and understanding for the wisdom behind it.

Visualization: Close your eyes. Be in the stillness for a couple of seconds so you feel grounded and centered.

When you feel ready, let your body sink into your sadness, your grief, as much as you can. Dedicate these few short moments to giving all of your attention to the sense of grief that lives within you.

See the grief as sandbags. They sit on your shoulders, on your heart, around your hips. Sit in the heaviness of grief.

And at the same time you are sinking into your grief, invite a part of you to move out from underneath the heavy grief bags and become neutral. Look at the grief that your body has taken on; look close at the effects on your body. Notice how it manifests. As the observer, take some time to remove the sandbags from all the places they are resting on, if you believe there is too much weight or discomfort. Each time you remove one, notice the lightness in your body.

Cast all the sand from the bags into an ocean that you visualize. Imagine all the particulates of sand are rejoined with their home in the ocean, which also represents the entirety of emotions. Water equals emotion. Grief is not a linear feeling. As you stand by the ocean shore, let your body sway to the rhythm of the ocean waves. Think of how grief moves through you in waves, sometimes catapulting you and crashing you, and then bringing you to a peaceful feeling. Focus on the moments of peace that you are able to savor. Absorb as much of the peace and feeling of surrender that the ocean waves embody as you can. Find refuge in the stillness.

With a calm state of mind, walk back into the body that you removed yourself from temporarily. This time, put your gaze deep within the spirals of your heart. Travel through the layers of the heart to find the part of it that is electrical energy. You may see this electrical energy as streaks of blue. And within the electric layer, notice if you have any long projections or cords of energy that are extending out from you like live wires. Maybe they extend out to someone you are no longer in contact with, to a deceased pet, or to losses you experienced as a child, like friends you left behind. Energetically, if we are trying to connect with loved ones that have passed or situations that have ended, we end up feeding our energy into "sinkholes," and we become depleted and drained.

So what you can try now is to first put caps on all those live wires, so your energy flow is no longer being directed out and dissipated. Once you have done this, roll each energy cord in towards your heart, folding it over and over on top of itself until it reaches your heart. And when it arrives, let this coil of energy go right to the center of your heart. See how vibrant your heart becomes when you harness this energy. Do this for all the cords that are outstretched, capping them and rolling them in to your heart. Feel a boost of energy in your heart because of all the energy flux that you have just created. This uplifting energy further removes any blocks or heaviness from your body as a result of the effects of grieving.

Now that you have completed the visualization, come back fully to the present moment. Rest both your hands on your heart and open your eyes.

Meditation: Meditate on the relationship between your heart and lungs. See them as working together, united and positive, beating and breathing in harmony. Together they are stronger than any force in the external world. Sit in honor and gratitude for this team that supports you and releases you from any suppressive grief.

Grounding (Feeling Ungrounded or Detached From Life)

Physical description: The symptoms of a person who is not grounded will manifest as fatigue, a feeling of being worn out, and dissociation from life. Often, ungrounded people will appear spacey, with a certain overlay of emptiness and an inability to stay in the present moment while performing their daily activities.

Energy center(s): Root, solar plexus

Nourishment: *Diet*—(1) Eat high-quality protein from animal sources (e.g., lean, organic meats; eggs; low-fat cheeses) or vegetable sources (e.g., legumes, nuts, seeds); (2) Eat small, frequent meals to keep blood sugar stabilized; (3) Eat with hands food not normally eaten with hands, to ensure a body-food connection; (4) Try eating on the ground or floor to emphasize the body-earth-food relationship; (5) Emphasize foods grown in the earth, such as yams, sweet potatoes, and beets; (6) Eat red-colored foods to energize the root chakra. *Supplements*—(1) Protein powder supplement (rice, soy, whey); (2) Mineral supplement for fortifying body structure and function like bone density.

Emotion(s): Anxiety, inadequacy, distrust, feeling threatened, insecurity about one's existence

Limiting belief(s): I do not belong. I do not exist. Life is a struggle.

Power animal: Buffalo

Flower essence(s): Angelica, Baby Blue Eyes, California Pitcher Plant, Gorse, Rosemary

Affirmation(s): I embrace and value my connection to this earthly realm. My life is real and true. I live fully and completely. I am rooted to my existence. I am present. I am.

Visualization: Close your eyes and watch your breath. Is it shallow? Does your breath travel into the depths of your belly? Are you breathing rapidly, or is your breath pacing nicely with the rest of your body?

Become blanketed in full awareness. Use your breath as your vehicle to discover how aware you are. Accept the current form of your breath. See it as artistry. Allow it to glide down to your low belly, like a heavy anchor dropping to the ocean floor. As your breath reaches your belly, you feel a sense of aliveness coming over you. Your entire body, especially your legs and feet, start to prickle with the joy of being fully human and in the present moment.

Feel the warm prickles in the base of your spine. Concentrate them until you feel a warm sensation in your low back. This feeling of warmth infuses you with a sense of safety and security. You release any fear through your breathing. Imagine that you plant a small seed in your low-back area, and it begins to grow quickly. This is the seed of your life. You see the seed sprouting and strengthening itself in your low back. It grows and sprouts long, tenacious tendrils that travel down your legs. They wrap themselves firmly around your thighs, knees, calves, and feet. You feel secure and not confined, as the tendrils are infinitely strong, but also very flexible.

You can go where you need to be. The green extensions of your life seed burrow deep into the soil of the earth underneath your feet and travel down into the heart of the earth, pulsing at the center of the planet. The earth welcomes your life and secures your life's tendrils within her. At once, you feel safe and protected, completely grounded and alive.

Your breath continues to ride you into the present moment. You sense a tingling sensation in your legs and feet that you have not experienced before. You feel their strength and ability to take you forward on your path. You wiggle your fingers and your feet and open your eyes to your new, vibrant life ahead!

Meditation: Meditate while standing up, and envision that you have roots going from your feet deep into the earth. Focus on the connection you have with your feet and with the earth.

Give yourself a foot rub or treat yourself to one from someone else.

Guilt

Physical description: A feeling arising from internal conflict about how one acted or didn't act in a situation and how that action or lack of it may have ultimately (directly or indirectly) caused harm to others.

Energy center(s): Root, sacral, solar plexus, heart, throat, third eye, crown

Nourishment: Become aware of and release any guilt that arises from eating certain foods or from eating in general.

Emotion(s): Worry, regret, anxiety, depression, shame

Limiting belief(s): I am ultimately responsible for everyone's happiness. It's my fault this happened. Others' opinions of me matter significantly, sometimes even more than my own.

Power animal: Coyote

Flower essence(s): Aspen, Filaree, Heather, Pine

Affirmation(s): I take ownership for my actions. I am free from entanglements that serve me incorrectly. I value my judgment. I stand my ground.

Visualization: Visualize your body from a short distance, using your third eye vision. See how all the guilt you have accumulated has manifested itself in your physical body. The guilt you feel appears as a cloud of dirt around you, barely impenetrable. When you scan your body to look at your feet, you notice they are mired in mud, and you are stuck, unable to move. Guilt has put your life on hold; it has you in its grip of fear and shame, and you see your body sinking deeper and deeper with each feeling of guilt that gets added to the mass of mud. Let's morph the guilt into something that will suit your life better.

Gaze up at the sky and ask for some clearing rain to shower down upon you. Observe the cloud that journeys to just over your head, about six feet above, and begins to release warm, tiny rain droplets. These raindrops are not ordinary; they contain the ability to clear you from all guilt and all emotions associated with the guilt. As the droplets move the presence of guilt through your energy field and body, at first, you notice streaks of clarity set forth by the paths of hundreds of tiny water droplets. As the rain continues to fall, with some momentum, you see the guilt wash away. Other emotions, like shame and fear, are layered underneath the grime of guilt. These, too, begin to be removed from your being, falling away into the puddle of water collecting at your feet.

Once your field and body are clear and clean, focus on your feet. They are movable now, as the water has created more fluidity within the mud. You pick up each foot individually and step on to the neighboring patch of green grass. Now you rest on firm, solid ground covered with fresh, bright green grass. Seeing the green color makes your heart swell with hope, confidence, and acceptance. Your energy field is now crystal clear and completely free from any guilt dirt or debris. Surround your being with a protective quartz pyramidal structure.

And when you are ready, extend your consciousness back into your being fully and completely. Feel the sense of renewal and joy of life running through your circulatory and nervous systems. Mentally affirm, "I am free!"

Meditation: In a meditative space, focus on the event that prompted your feelings of guilt. When you go back to that moment, how does your body respond?

Now go back to that same moment and transform the outcome. Keep that image in your mind's eye and feel the corresponding feeling in your body.

Now envision what you can do to let go of your guilt. Come up with at least three solutions. The next time you feel guilt creeping in, snap your fingers several times to give you the energetic space to create a new baseline and re-envision the situation.

Gum Disease (Periodontitis, Periodontal Disease)

Physical description: The mucosal lining in the mouth that keeps the teeth protected becomes infected or prone to receding to the base of tooth, which can ultimately cause tooth loss.

Energy center(s): Root, heart, throat

Nourishment: *Diet*—(1) Reduce or avoid refined sugars (found primarily in processed foods); (2) Eat proportionally greater amount of fiber-rich foods (such as nonstarchy vegetables, legumes, whole grains); (3) Throughout the day, consume green tea for its anti-inflammatory and antioxidant benefits. *Supplements*—(1) Vitamin C to support the immune system and maintain the integrity of gum tissue; (2) A high-quality multivitamin and mineral containing vitamin A (or beta-carotene), zinc, vitamin E, and folic acid; (3) Coenzyme Q10, a potent antioxidant and nutrient to assist in energy production; (4) A probiotic supplement to help restore gut flora in mucosal membranes such as those in the mouth.

Emotion(s): Insecurity, frustration, anger

Limiting belief(s): I am exposed; my foundation is coming apart. Unspoken words wear on me. I hold within me valuable truth that I am afraid to reveal. I am becoming detached from others.

Power animal: Raven

Flower essence(s): Corn, Heather, Saguaro, Scleranthus

Affirmation(s): I sit comfortably within my authentic self. I am free to be me and to speak my mind and heart. I am open to sharing my thoughts, opinions, and beliefs with others in a way that serves my highest good. I am solid and secure in myself. I accept and love my roots and origins.

Visualization: *This visualization works best if you actually use a glass of water and walk through the activities mentioned.*

In your hands you hold a glass filled with the purest water possible. With the flow of your breath, see currents of energy traveling from your hands into the glass. You invite the energy of the sun to grace this water. And from the sky spills forth lavish sunlight, which cascades down into this glass. The water becomes imbued with the radiance of the sun and all of the healing carried in the sun's infinite, golden rays. You can feel the yang energy of the sun pulsing up through your arms and into your chest, traveling into your heart. You thank the sun for its contribution, and it disappears back into the sky.

You continue to hold the glass very carefully as you breathe in to call forth the energy of the moon. With your beckoning, the moon appears before you, full and sparkling, blanketing you in an iridescent, glittering light that feels cool and comforting. With this silvery light, you can feel your creative energy surfacing and opening to expression. You welcome this light with a deep appreciation. At once, the moonlight pours into and mixes with the sun-infused water.

Together, the sun and moon energies harmoniously swirl together in the water. As they spiral and move dynamically together, you call in the energy of the rainbow—all the healing colors of red, orange, yellow, green, blue, and violet. They pour into your water, circulating through it several times. The rainbow returns to its source.

In your hands, you are holding a healing elixir composed of the healing energies of the sun, moon, and rainbow. This potentiated water has the ability to create healing alchemy in your body. You notice you are very thirsty, and you slowly take a sip of this water. You hold it in your mouth, first letting it fill your mouth. You can feel the aliveness of the sun, the creativity of the moon, and the vibrancy of the rainbow come alive within your mouth, coating the inner walls of your mouth, soaking your gums and mucosal-tissue lining. At once, your gum tissue feels healed, soothed, and rejuvenated.

You swallow the liquid and allow it to travel down your esophagus and into your stomach. The liquid carries through this passage a healing ribbon of these golden, silvery, and multicolored energies.

You take another sip of the liquid, again letting its healing vibration circulate throughout your mouth. Your gum tissue responds to the dynamic circulation of the universal energies. Whenever you feel it's the right time, you swallow the liquid, feeling the energies dancing along the tube within you and coalescing into your stomach, filling it with health and healing.

With the last sip, you savor the sun, moon, and rainbow energies by tasting them on your tongue, and then you allow this divine mixture to coat your teeth and gum tissue. You swallow it slowly and watch its healing energies line the way to your stomach.

Your take your hands from the glass and reach them to the sky in gratitude to the elements that have helped you to heal everything from mouth to stomach. The fine, mucosal lining is now strong and supported. Your teeth shine with the energy of the moon, and your gums hold them securely.

Meditation: Every night before going to sleep, journal about the things you wished you had said that day. Ask for insight from your third eye about the realm of reasons for not saying them. For example, was there fear or anger involved? During meditation, open your mind to ideas about how you can get your message across in a creative way that you feel comfortable about. Log these ideas in your journal.

Hair Loss (Alopecia Areata, Baldness)

Physical description: Excessive loss of hair from the scalp, which can be due to a variety of causes, including heredity, hormonal shifts (e.g., pregnancy, menopause), illness, blood sugar imbalance, iron deficiency, and pharmaceuticals, to name a few.

Energy center(s): Root, crown

Nourishment: *Diet*—(1) Reduce or avoid refined sugar (typically found in processed foods); (2) Emphasize high-quality protein, such as legumes, lean meats, eggs, and low-fat cheeses; (3) If iron deficient, eat iron-rich foods, such as lean meats, black beans, and dark green, leafy vegetables. *Supplements*—(1) A high-quality multivitamin and mineral that contains the entire B complex, as well as vitamins C and E and zinc; (2) An iron supplement if iron deficient; (3) Biotin; (4) Silica (from horsetail herb).

Emotion(s): Fear, anxiety, feeling overwhelmed

Limiting belief(s): My spirit is weak. I want to escape. I am losing it! I am so frustrated I could pull my hair out! I am stressed and ready to blow my top!

Power animal: Lion

Flower essence(s): Cherry Plum, Lavender

Affirmation(s): I am calm and soothed by knowing that all happens with divine perfection. I sit in the throne of understanding, wearing a crown of beauty studded with gems of trust.

Visualization: Close your eyes and give yourself permission to sink into the present moment completely and fully.

Envision before you three vials. The first vial is filled with a golden, viscous liquid the consistency of warm honey. It contains plant oils that are known to nourish your scalp. You open the delicate vial and pour forth its contents into the palm of your hands. You distribute this radiant, vibrant liquid into both palms, and then you gently and intentionally move your hands to the front of your scalp, permitting enough time for this resinous elixir to saturate the pores on top of your head. Then you move your hands back over your scalp incrementally, so every square inch of your scalp has been covered with the soft, healing salve. Each of the thousands of hair follicles on your head is bathed in this precious liquid.

You take a deep breath in, and as you do so, the glistening liquid follows your breath by moving even further into your scalp. With another breath, it circulates around your scalp, providing it with the raw essence it needs to promote healthy hair growth. Once the golden liquid has been completely absorbed by the hair follicles and scalp, they are shining and luminescent with the vibrant energy of youth.

You then pick up the second vial, which contains a liquid that is emerald green. The information you receive on this vial is that it is a complex infusion of vital plant energy that will strengthen your hair and follicles. You pour the liquid from the vial directly on top of your scalp, and its silky smoothness coats the entire scalp and every single hair on your head. You feel an invigorating sensation on your scalp, a menthol-feeling, minty richness that makes every hair on your head come alive. Every hair on your head immediately becomes enriched and thickened by the presence of the plant material, which supplies important strengthening compounds. Each hair spirals with its own long thread of this liquid. The essence of the hair dances with the plant energy, and the plant energy coils down from each hair strand, making its way into the earth. The connection with the earth results in healing energy of love and growth to be infused into each tendril of plant energy. They glow with the green light of growth, and this light pulses up the coil back to your head to feed the hairs. As you take a deep breath in, the plant energy becomes embedded into the matrix of every hair and every hair yet to be, which reside dormant under the scalp.

You pick up the third and last vial, and you see that it contains a pinkish, radiant essential oil combination derived from flowers. There are only ten drops of liquid in this tiny bottle, and the information on the vial tells you that you need to evenly spread the drops over your scalp, with three towards the front, three in the middle, three towards the back, and one at the nape of your neck. You begin to apply the drops as was directed, and the wisdom you receive from these flower-derived essential oils is that they will protect your scalp from any damage from the environment, including pollution, toxins, and stress. They require that you provide them with healthy food from your diet. The essential oils set in place a boundary of protection and love to ensure that your hair stays blossoming and beautiful.

Once you've applied the aromatic oils, a wave of calm washes over you. And you take in the calm feeling with your breath as you inhale fully and then exhale, as though you were riding the wave of peace.

Meditation: Every day, meditate on the crown of your head and visualize your hair growing, like seeds growing in a garden. Affirm, "My hair grows thickly, quickly, and evenly."

To support this exercise, plant seeds (like barley grass or wheat grass, which resemble hair strands) and, with intention, nourish their growth.

Hammertoes (See Foot Pain)

Headaches (See also Migraines)

Physical description: Pain in the head or upper neck that can occur in many different forms (e.g., migraine, tension, or cluster headaches) and as the result of varied causes.

Energy center(s): Third eye, crown

Nourishment: *Diet*—(1) Work with a qualified healthcare professional to identify food allergies; (2) Minimize or eliminate foods high in amines, such as chocolate, cheese, alcoholic beverages, shellfish, and citrus fruits; (3) Avoid foods laden in certain food additives (e.g., sulfites, nitrates, nitrites, monosodium glutamate, artificial sweeteners); (4) Remove caffeine-containing foods and beverages; (5) Eat small, frequent meals throughout the day to keep blood sugar balanced; (6) Reduce animal-based products, particularly meats, as they contain relatively high amounts of an inflammatory fatty acid (arachidonic acid); (7) Eat foods high in anti-inflammatory fats, such as fish, flaxseed oil, leafy greens, and nuts; (8) Incorporate garlic and ginger for their anti-inflammatory properties; (9) Drink adequate fluids to keep hydrated. *Supplements*—(1) Magnesium to help promote healthy nerve-cell and blood-vessel function; (2) B-complex vitamin to assist in the breakdown of histamine in foods and to ensure adequate energy production; (3) Coenzyme Q10 for healthy energy production; (4) Botanicals such as butterbur, ginger, and feverfew; (5)

5-hydroxytryptophan for elevating levels of serotonin (a neurotransmitter) and endorphins.

Emotion(s): Anger, fear, worry

Limiting belief(s): My head aches with the pressures of everyday living. I cannot escape from thoughts that create tension and worry.

Power animal: Peacock

Flower essence(s): Iris, Lavender, Mimulus, Nasturtium, Peppermint, Star of Bethlehem, White Chestnut

Affirmation(s): My mind is quiet and free of overwhelming thoughts. My inner journey takes me from my head into my heart. My thoughts liberate my true self into a realm of creativity. My head is calm and collects ideas, opinions, and thoughts that serve me and others.

Visualization: A large wooden box with a glass door appears before you, and you decide to open the door and step in. The space inside is rather small and would only fit two people comfortably. There is a small wooden bench inside, and you take a seat. As you breathe in deeply, you notice that the space around you begins to get warm. You breathe in the warm air, letting it fall down to your belly to warm the fire within you.

You sit in the silence, and with another couple of breaths, you are engulfed in a heat that penetrates your muscles and tissues very deeply. The heat feels completely comfortable and soothing. Your body absorbs the infrared heat through every inch of the surface area of your skin. Another couple of breaths, and you break a light sweat. Looking down at your skin, you see beads of water dotting your arms, chest, and legs. The healing smells of eucalyptus and lavender waft through the air. You breathe them in with the intention of invigorating your mind and brain and removing any blocks.

The sweat continues to bubble up through your pores, and you have the realization that you are releasing more than just sweat, or water. Every pore has expelled any limiting beliefs, outdated opinions, or patterns that hold you back. There is a free feeling that washes over you from this sweat. You feel cleansed from within; the repetition of thoughts in your mind has now been broken. You are the master of your mind, and at a deep level, you have decided to let any tension in your body melt away into the dewdrops on your skin. Your blood vessels are open wide to allow for increased circulation and healing within you. The level of minerals in your body, like calcium and magnesium, are now brought back into balance.

You grab on to the towel hanging on the wall and begin wiping off, from the top of your body to the bottom, all the sweat, which has gathered your pains, past, and patterns that prevent you from progressing. The towel is soaking wet after a couple of seconds, and your body is comfortably dry, smooth, and silky.

Your attention is brought back to the breath, and as you focus there, the infrared heat starts to dissipate. The box you are sitting in becomes cooler and more refreshing with each breath. You feel incredibly balanced; the yin and yang elements within you are in equal measure. At last, you sit surrounded by room temperature. After a couple of seconds, you decide to open the glass door and step outside. Your headache is gone; your body is healed.

Meditation: Meditate on your head. Envision it completely littered with excessive thoughts, stress, and unrealized ideas and dreams. Now see your mind let go of all the excesses, one by one, emptying itself out, like a suitcase. After the meditation, make a conscious effort to scrutinize everything you put into the suitcase of your mind.

Hearing Loss

Physical description: The complete or partial inability to discern sounds.

Energy center(s): Throat

Nourishment: *Supplements*—(1) Magnesium; (2) Folic acid.

Emotion(s): Irritation, denial, apathy

Limiting belief(s): I tune out messages. I am deaf to the cries around me.

Power animal: Mouse

Flower essence(s): Cosmos, Star Tulip

Affirmation(s): I am in tune with healing sounds. I resonate with my self and my environment. I listen to the sounds and signs of the universe.

Visualization: Sit comfortably in a relatively quiet area. Let all of your senses except for hearing dissolve in the moment. Refrain from tasting, close your eyes, let go of anything you are touching with your hands, and ignore any smells wafting your way. Give your full focus in these next few moments to only your sense of hearing.

Transform your body into one large organ of hearing. Rather than hearing with just your ears, extend your sense of hearing into every part of you, so that every single cell is listening to the subtle sounds around you. Imagine your skin cells absorbing the texture of sound that surrounds you like a blanket, the cells of your digestive tract ingesting sounds and processing them, the cells of the nervous system responding to the subtle vibration of sounds you are enveloped in. There are sounds you may not have heard before, and you allow them to engulf you like a wave. You may receive and process the sounds visually, as shapes or figures; they may conjure up certain emotions, bring you back to the past, or transport you to the future. Simply observe as much as you can in the next minute. Let the multitude layers of sound cascade into your being. Peel away anything from within—any blocks, stagnation, or old hurts—that obstructs or interferes with the sounds around you, so everything becomes transparent. Sounds become amplified as you peel away the barriers. Although the presence of sound in your environment has become magnified, it feels comforting. You sit comfortably in receptivity.

Now shift your awareness away from every cell in your body to your ears, imagining they morph into large conch shells, extending outward from the head. Your conch-shell ears are clear and connected to sounds from far away, as well as those that are near. The spiraled structure of the shell keeps the layers of different sounds distinct even in the midst of a flurry of noise.

Envision clear, watery, aquamarine-colored energy entering the top of your head and funneling through your ears, moving through the spiral of the conch shells before exiting. This energy clears your ears from obstruction, giving you the ability to hear divine guidance, your instinct and intuition, along with your voice of truth.

Now shift your imagination to that of a fountain of green light coming up from your heart. This light follows a trajectory upwards and curves to flow through your ears, filling them with love, compassion, and giving and receiving in equal measure. Your ability to hear has become fine-tuned through the movement of these energies through you.

After this visualization, continue to practice listening as much as possible. By exercising it, you will strengthen your ability.

Meditation: Journal on the following: What messages have you heard loud and clear? What have you been tuning out?

Allow yourself to be in nature at least one time per week, and practice sitting and listening to the layers of sounds filling your ears.

Heart Disease

Physical description: *Heart disease,* in general, refers to any number of heart and blood-vessel abnormalities, including a buildup of plaque, which can lead to a heart attack (blocked blood flow and oxygen to the heart) or to chest pain (sometimes referred to as angina).

Energy center(s): Heart

Nourishment: *Diet*—(1) Eat a Mediterranean-style diet high in fresh vegetables, lean protein (preferably fish), healthy oils (olive, flaxseed, canola), whole grains, nuts, seeds, and legumes; Mediterranean heart-healthy favorites include tomatoes for their lycopene content, pomegranate for its antioxidant activity, and garlic for its ability to promote healthy blood vessels and blood fats; (2) Avoid processed foods high in trans fat, saturated fat (typically animal foods), and refined sugars. *Supplements*—(1) A high-quality multivitamin and mineral that includes vitamins C and E and the entire B complex; (2) Omega-3 fatty acids (preferably from fish oil) to reduce inflammation and balance blood fats; (3) Magnesium for improving blood flow (oxygen) to the heart; (4) Niacin and arginine for healthy blood-vessel function. (Note: you may encounter skin flushing with niacin use.)

Emotion(s): Hurt, grief, anger, separation, fear of intimacy

Limiting belief(s): I am not loved. I am not nourished by the flow of love and life. There are blocks to my receiving and giving love. Love causes pain. I am disconnected from a source of love.

Power animal: Lion

Flower essence(s): Bleeding Heart, Borage, Calendula, Evening Primrose, Holly, Mimulus, Zinnia

Affirmation(s): I am full of love and joy. Love extends through me and is received by me in equal measure. I am open and free to accepting love in my life. Love flows through my heart and blood vessels. My heart blossoms in the rays of life and holds the nectar of bliss.

Visualization: Start in the place of your heart, centered in the middle of your chest. Crystallize all of your attention in this space. Notice your heart space. Feel if there is any congestion or blocks or if blood flows freely through it.

Now see your heart as a gigantic rose, filled with layers of velvet pink petals. See the petals multiply and extend out even further. Imagine yourself as a bumblebee looking upon this gorgeous rose with delight, seeing all its sweetness. See yourself as the bee traversing through the labyrinthine layers of petals, feeling the gentle texture of the petals as you pass through them, soaking in the sweet smell.

Eventually, you funnel into the core of the heart rose. In the heart center, it is very quiet, and the space feels expansive and vast. You feel at home here and lie down to rest. Breathing in deeply, you sink into this beautiful space. You have not been here in a long time, and you have been missed. From the stillness, the heart energy calls you to help create flowing smoothness and softness throughout its structure. You are honored by the request to help this amazing heart energy, who has a regal feel, like a king or a queen. Your protective nature springs into action, and, as a bee, you spiral through the rose, collecting all debris, blocks, and stagnation from the rose.

At the very end of your journey, you have accumulated many blocks that appear as old memories, hurts, emotions, losses, and traumas. You bundle them up and fly high up to the sky to release them, and as they float back down to the rose, they begin to transform to nourishing drops of water that sprinkle the rose petals. The rose extends its petals further with love for the water. The water winds its way into and out of the rose, bringing it the life force it needs and then moving on, like the river of blood nourishing the heart. The shower of pure water continues, cleansing the rose petals, creating a flow to purify and clear the heart from all other residue. At last, the rose is clean, clear, and pure, and is able to extend its petals to all life, in healthy giving and receiving. The heart takes in only that which is for its highest good and extends in service only to the limit that it feels comfortable. The rose fills with compassion and love. And the bee watches over it to ensure that it is always protected from harm.

Breathe in gently through your heart space, softly ruffling the petals of your heart with the inhale. And on the exhale, see a vibrant green glow over the space of your heart, sealing in all the clearing and protection you have received.

Meditation: See your heart as a royal throne. Who is your internal ruler? A benevolent queen? A cantankerous king? An innocent princess?

Open another dimension of your heart as you circle within its spiral caverns. Expand into your essence. Be here for a couple of minutes, enjoying the feeling of freedom.

Heartburn (Esophageal Reflux, Ulcers, Stomach Problems)

Physical description: A painful, burning sensation felt in the region of the stomach.

Energy center(s): Solar plexus

Nourishment: *Diet*—(1) Avoid fatty, fried foods, citrus fruits and juices, caffeinated foods and beverages (coffee, tea, chocolate), tomatoes, and spicy foods, especially before bedtime; (2) Eat small, frequent meals throughout the day rather than large ones; (3) Chew food thoroughly and take sufficient time to eat; (4) Drink adequate water in between meals; (5) Drink herbal teas, such as chamomile, licorice, and mint; (6) Work with a qualified healthcare professional to identify food allergies. *Supplements*—(1) A mineral supplement containing calcium and magnesium; (2) Digestive enzymes (but no hydrochloric acid) with meals.

Emotion(s): Anger, rage, "burning up," fear

Limiting belief(s): I become enraged by the turbulence around me. I can't digest in all the irritation. I am overflowing with acidic anger.

Power animal: Beaver

Flower essence(s): Black Cohosh, Chamomile, Dill, Rabbitbrush, Shasta Daisy

Affirmation(s): I keep my life in perspective. Harmony is threaded through the fabric of my life. The big picture of my life is integrated with my everyday actions.

Visualization: Imagine you are sitting at a simple wooden table. You are relaxed and focused on your breathing. Pay special attention to your stomach. Send some deep breaths of fresh air into the pocket of the stomach to prepare it for this clearing visualization.

Before you, on the table, sit two small glasses filled with liquid. You are intrigued by their contents, and you feel that they are there for you to heal any issues that you are having with heartburn. One glass feels like it is available to heal your emotional issues around heartburn, while the other is to help you with the physical manifestation.

The first glass is filled with an opaque liquid that looks similar to milk, yet it is opalescent. When you look closely at it, you notice a swirling mixture of light pastel streams of color embedded into the milky matrix. You take a sip, and it tastes good. So you drink the entire contents in one swallow. The swirling, milky liquid winds down your throat, through your esophagus, and finally into your stomach. It coats all these parts of you and penetrates into the tissue a bit, releasing any stuck fear and replacing that fear with nurturing and a soothing feel. The doorway entering your stomach, which is typically tight and constrained, is especially coated and imbued with the message of peace. This milky liquid sends the energy of "Everything will be all right" to your stomach on a very deep level.

And, in an instant, you have the recognition that you are confronted only with situations you can handle. Nothing seems insurmountable. You feel cradled and supported, yet empowered and invigorated at the same time. All the fears that you were trying to digest are now relieved. Your stomach is relaxed and able to look at these situations in a larger context. You remove yourself from the worry embedded into your stomach.

You are then ready to take in the second liquid, which is a yellowish fluid that looks something like lemonade. Already, as the glass sits in your hands, you have a feeling of joy that washes over you. There is something very pleasant about this fluid. You take a sip, and it tastes sweet and tangy. This small sip of liquid journeys to your stomach, and along the way, it quells any inflammation. You take the remaining sips. This liquid contains the consciousness of balance, and the mere presence of it in your stomach sends a message to harmonize the acid production and distribution. This added energy washes through you, and you feel a sense of relief. Your stomach no longer feels like a volcano, spewing forth acid with stress or with meals. It now feels like it has been taken care of and provided with support for clearing and release. Take a deep breath and send this second liquid down to your stomach, swirling it together with the first in your stomach.

Place your hands on your stomach, and ask that your healer and warrior energies work with your stomach from this point forward to digest life's experiences without undue stress, worry, or inflammation.

Meditation: Engage in a sipping meditation, in which you use a glass of water (about eight ounces). With every sip, you think of a word that would help you to flow more with the river of life. Think of the word, take a sip of water, and see that intention filling your belly with the ability to synthesize, integrate, and fully participate without fear in all of life's events. Continue until the glass is empty.

Hemorrhoids

Physical description: Swollen, protruding veins from inside the rectum or outside the anus that may bleed or cause pain or discomfort.

Energy center(s): Root

Nourishment: *Diet*—(1) Eat a fiber-rich diet, including skin-on fruits and vegetables (carrots, beets, apples, pears). Broccoli, legumes, peas, whole grains, and berries are excellent choices; (2) Drink adequate water/liquids; (3) Ensure adequate healthy, liquid omega-3 fats (e.g., flaxseed oil, canola oil) intake to reduce inflammation and to lubricate the mucosal lining of the gut. *Supplements*—(1) Reduce inflammation by taking an omega-3 oil supplement (from flaxseed or fish oil); (2) Incorporate a fiber supplement, such as one with oat bran, psyllium, apple pectin, or guar gum; (3) Take a vitamin C and bioflavonoid supplement (e.g., hesperidin) to help with maintaining healthy blood vessels.

Emotion(s): Anger, fury, stagnation, inflammation, fear, insecurity

Limiting belief(s): I am angry that I have to let go. I fear completion. Letting go is a struggle. Moving on from the past feels unsafe and risky.

Power animal: Polar bear

Flower essence(s): Angel's Trumpet, Blackberry, Elm, Honeysuckle, Sagebrush

Affirmation(s): Beginnings and ends are part of nature, and I accept both in my life. I painlessly let go. I welcome completion. My body, mind, and spirit shift from stagnation into seamless, fluid action. I release burdens and expectations.

Visualization: Close your eyes and swallow in some deep breaths to center and ground you. Let the air of your breath lift your consciousness up and out of your body, giving yourself a view of your body from just a couple of feet above it. Imagine your physical body rests on a bed of soft, cushioned, cloudlike substance. As you know, the physical body is like a filter, and it can collect memories, events, thought patterns, and emotional clusters, if we do not process them. Sometimes, it becomes difficult to release one or all of these. It can take time, and if the body wants you to remove these, it may present you with symptoms, like hemorrhoids. Hemorrhoids let your body know that there is something you need to dispose of—something that may be tied to something inflammatory.

So begin by scanning your body to see where there are challenges to letting go of something. In particular, examine your colon. Your colon travels up the right side of your abdomen, across it, and then down the left side, ending in the rectum. Use your special intuitive sight to look inside your colon, your organ that helps you to let go and surrender, to see whether there are things that have become trapped inside. If you notice some objects or images, acknowledge them without judgment.

You are then presented with a glass jug containing sparkling, cool water. Pour this shining, bluish, healing water into the colon, and let it stream all the way through until the end. The water carries with it everything you wish to remove from your colon, including any inflammation, physical and emotional. And when it pours out of you from your rectum, let it release through the cloud your body is laying on and become like rain. This rain contains everything you are letting go of, and it falls to the earth below you. The earth takes in these droplets, transforms what you have let go of into healing, and recycles this water to re-enter your colon. A constant cycle of water fluxing through your colon, being sent to the earth, and then coming back from the earth to your colon continues for a couple of seconds until your colon feels clean, cool, and clear.

See your body as a part of nature, with a built-in cycle of receiving and letting go. Restore this healthy cycle in your body through your intention. And when you have finished, direct your consciousness back into your body, become yourself fully, and awaken.

Meditation: For one week, focus on consciously letting go of a past event, person, or item, or of something or someone that you feel plagues you in the present. Practice doing so by writing (but not sending) letters to the person in question, donating the items to charity, or by gently working towards undoing a painful habit that you have found yourself stuck to (like eating a poor diet or not exercising).

Hepatitis (SEE LIVER PROBLEMS)

Herpes Simplex Virus (SEE VIRAL INFECTION, VENEREAL DISEASE)

High Blood Cholesterol (SEE HYPERCHOLESTEROLEMIA)

High Blood Sugar (SEE HYPERGLYCEMIA)

Hives (Urticaria)

Physical description: White, pink, or reddish raised bumps or patches on the skin that form in response to allergies, stress, changes in temperature, the application of pressure, and/or exercise, to name a few causes.

Energy center(s): Root

Nourishment: *Diet*—(1) Avoid food additives, such as dyes, artificial sweeteners, and preservatives (e.g., BHA, BHT, sulfites); (2) Work with a qualified healthcare professional to determine food allergies; (3) Avoid typical food allergens: dairy, shellfish, eggs, soy, nuts, and gluten. *Supplements*—(1) Vitamin C and bioflavonoids like quercetin to increase the breakdown of histamine.

Emotion(s): Defensiveness, insecurity, shyness

Limiting belief(s): I am under attack. My sensitivity makes it difficult to be in harmony with my self and the environment. I overreact. Life gets under my skin and irritates me.

Power animal: Bee

Flower essence(s): Corn, Larch, Pink Monkeyflower, Yarrow

Affirmation(s): I am congruent in my inner feelings and outer approach to living. I sip and savor the nectar of life in my everyday routine. The environment comforts and nurtures me.

Visualization: Close your eyes and visualize your entire body surrounded by several layers of gold, extending at least six feet outside of your physical body, expanding in all directions. You are completely encapsulated by this protective sheath, which resembles a beehive. Within the golden hive, your physical body is assembled with the complexity of a well-designed honeycomb. Each system is a structurally organized unit, and all layers fold upon themselves to give you your perfectly functioning body.

Make your consciousness very small and enter a tiny pore found on your skin. In this space, what opens up to you is the complete landscape of your skin, which you are invited to explore in a fluid, floating fashion, as if you were a honeybee. Gliding from above, you begin at your head and neck area, scanning for any sites of inflammation or itching. If you observe any, you are able to invoke the assistance of the team of bees, or your immune system messengers, who arrive to the area to coat it with liquid honey, or the protective life-force energy within the body. See in your mind's eye that the areas—on your face, neck, chest, and even upper back—have absorbed the soothing liquid honey into the honeycomb structure of the cells.

Once you have coated these areas, move your honeybee awareness, buzzing to the beat of your breath, to your low back and belly, paying attention to any areas that are affected by itching hives, welts, or shingles. In this areas, shine the liquid light of the golden honey in these places, making them calm and quiet, relieving any eruptions in the honeycomb of the skin. With the buzz of your breath, see the liquid, golden honey saturate your legs, starting from the top and drizzling through to the bottom. Every cell, or honeycomb, is glowing with peace. There is no more irritation. The army of your immune system, which you can visualize as a swarm of bees that live within your honeycomb, has dealt with any fires, battles, or invasions by coating them with the sweetness of their honey.

All the honey pours through your legs and pools at the bottom of your feet. Your feet feel soft and protected. Any negativity or problems that have made their way "under your skin" have now been sent to the bottoms of your feet, allowing them to slip out from your feet and into the ground, far away from you, into the molten liquid core of the earth. The earth naturally absorbs all these issues and burns away any pain, irritation, or fear.

When you are ready, zoom yourself out of the vehicle of the honeybee and let her join the rest of your vigilant immune system, carrying out the orders of your body. Move your awareness out of your body to the degree that you are able to look at your body and the surrounding space. Envision yourself as glowing, full of light, and all streams of energy are moving without obstruction within. You can see the inner workings of your immune system and skin as being in harmony, connecting through the liquid honey light that fills you.

Now take a gentle breath, breathing in the words "balance and protection." Make a subtle buzzing sound as you bring yourself back to the present moment.

Meditation: If you have hives, close your eyes and tune into the feeling you are experiencing. What is really getting under your skin? What does your instinct want you to react to?

Human Immunodeficiency Virus (HIV; SEE VIRAL INFECTION)

Hypercholesterolemia (High Blood Cholesterol)

Physical description: A buildup of the waxy, fatlike substance known as cholesterol in the arteries, causing reduced supply of oxygen and nutrients to tissues such as the heart.

Energy center(s): Heart

Nourishment: *Diet*—(1) Reduce or avoid your intake of animal foods (which are high in saturated fat and may increase blood cholesterol), such as meat and dairy products, and substitute fish or vegetable products (e.g., tofu); (2) Limit or avoid coffee, alcohol, excess sodium, and trans fat (the last two of which are found in processed foods); (3) Increase dietary soluble fiber by eating whole grains (e.g., barley, brown rice), legumes, nonstarchy vegetables, and fruits; (4) Use vegetable oils instead of solid fats; (5) Increase your consumption of garlic and onions. *Supplements*—(1) A soluble-fiber supplement (e.g., guar gum, apple pectin, psyllium) to help trap cholesterol in the gut and remove it from the body; (2) Niacin (Note: extreme facial flushing can occur when taking niacin.); (3) Garlic

Emotion(s): Stagnation, feeling overwhelmed, accumulation of feelings, withdrawal, feeling weighed down

Limiting belief(s): My life is full with challenges that block me from flowing freely. I am weighed down by stress. My heart's true feelings are left unexpressed.

Power animal: Hawk

Flower essence(s): Blackberry, Clematis, Walnut

Affirmation(s): I am clear of any and all interference in the river of life that runs through me. I am free, protected, and clear of stress and strain. I synthesize what is of value into the heart of my being.

Visualization: Close your eyes and with the power of your mind's eye, your internal vision, look into your body. Envision the intricate circulatory system as a series of roads; the main arteries are large roads with six lanes, smaller arteries are two-lane highways, veins are single-lane highways, and capillaries are intersections and roundabouts. If you were to see your body from a distance, it would appear as a detailed map of vasculature.

And now, looking within and from above, as if a tiny helicopter were carrying your consciousness, you ride through your body, looking for any road blocks, traffic accidents, cars off to the side of the road, or emergencies that need tending to. Start at the level of your head and weave your way through the labyrinth of vessels that line your brain. See whether there are any obstructions or a hint of damage or debris, and, if there are, use your internal speaker system to call attention to this area.

Call in the clean-up crews and emergency squads of the immune system. Make sure any obstruction has been cleared and then repaired by the internal teams, which repave roads and fix cars traveling on them. Take your time to survey the blocked area thoroughly, because if there is a block, it can be impacting the function of your brain. If there are any sites where cholesterol is piled up, send forth tiny pickup and dump trucks to remove the deposits and bring them back to the liver, so they can be packaged and sent out of the body. Guide your body through this process in the time it takes to do it thoroughly.

Once you feel confident that all roads are cleared of cholesterol debris, send a whole team of these cholesterol pickup and dump trucks throughout every inch of your internal highway of vessels.

Move through the neck, the upper body, and send a message out to recruit special trucks and workers to shovel the cholesterol out of the chambered highways weaving through the heart. All of the excess cholesterol gets dumped on to the trucks and sent back to the hub of the liver. Your liver thrives on this activity, packaging it into the bile so it can be released from the body. See the circulation of cholesterol moving through the liver, into the bile, and out through your intestines.

Keep that flow going while you continue with dispersing the cholesterol pickup vehicles throughout the body, this time through the abdomen and legs. Have a separate team of trucks moving at full speed through your arms and hands, picking up any sticky cholesterol debris.

As your body becomes cleared of cholesterol, you begin to feel more energy. Your mind opens up, your heart pumps more efficiently, and your blood vessels strengthen. Your breath moves to the beat of your heart. Hear your heart beating nice and rhythmically.

Now, in your helicopter, take yourself back to your liver. Steer your helicopter in circles over your liver, creating a whirlwind of activity that helps the liver remove any clogged structures from itself. This whirl of energy helps to balance the energy in the liver and prevent it from overproducing cholesterol. Affirm to your liver, "My body makes the perfect amount of cholesterol."

When you feel as though your liver is balanced, take your vehicle to the long tunnel of your small intestine. Place within your intestine tiny rafts of light that will capture any cholesterol that you eat and sail it out of the body, through the intestine. Your body has the wisdom to create more of these rafts of light as they are needed. You set an intention within your body and mind to be ever more mindful of the foods you eat, to ensure that you do not take in amounts of cholesterol and saturated fat that are not helpful for your body. You mentally program yourself to make conscious attempts to eat more plant foods—more vegetables, fruits, and grains—in place of animal foods.

And when you are ready, let your helicopter of vision travel to your third eye, where it lands. Its propeller quiets, its body remains still. You remain still, locked in the quiet moment. And at the moment of your choosing, open your eyes to your surroundings.

Meditation: In your living space, note accumulated items that seem to get in your way. Engage in a meditative clearing exercise by organizing, straightening, or purging items that no longer serve you.

Hyperglycemia (High Blood Sugar, Diabetes)

Physical description: The body is unable to efficiently process glucose (sugar) due to a lack of sufficient insulin from the pancreas, or from an inability of tissues to be sensitive to insulin's effects. As a result, glucose accumulates in the bloodstream, causing peripheral damage to nerves, eyes, skin, and red blood cells.

Energy center(s): Solar plexus

Nourishment: *Diet*—(1) Eat high-fiber, low-glycemic-index foods, such as legumes, whole grains, nonstarchy vegetables, and fruits; (2) Avoid simple sugars and processed foods high in saturated and trans fats. *Supplements*—(1) High-quality, high-potency multivitamin and mineral; (2) Chromium; (3) A fiber supplement; (4) Blood sugar balancing botanicals such as cinnamon, gymnema, fenugreek, and bitter melon; (5) Circulation-enhancing botanicals like bilberry, grapeseed extract, and ginkgo.

Emotion(s): Depletion, feeling overwhelmed, inadequacy

Limiting belief(s): It's never enough. My life has become routine. Stress pervades my everyday living. I am on overdrive to perform, and my expectations are high. I neglect myself.

Power animal: Hummingbird

Flower essence(s): Cherry Plum, Clematis, Dandelion, Evening Primrose, Hornbeam, Lady's Slipper, Mimulus, Sunflower, Zinnia

Affirmation(s): My life is saturated with sweetness. Life provides me with opportunities to become full with energy. My body organs are in harmony. I transform information from my environment into loving energy within. I embrace pleasure. My heart responds to joy.

Visualization: Take a few seconds to reflect on where you get the most joy in your life. Do you feel happy when you are working, when you are in the presence of family and friends, or while you are engaging in a sport or hobby? Do you perhaps have difficulty finding where the joy in your life is hiding?

See if you can crystallize one of those joyful moments, even if it's just a small spark. Hold it like a precious gem in your cupped hands. With the initiation of your inhale, imagine this tiny crystal pours forth a bountiful stream of a yellow-gold, honeylike substance—the essence of sweetness—into your hands. From this tiny morsel, you watch the abundant flow of sweetness being liberated from its intricate structure. You drink in this soft liquid energy through your mouth, and you watch it travel down into your digestive tract. It settles into your pancreas, which resides on the left side of your upper abdomen. Your pancreas soaks in this radiant, honeyed liquid, allowing it to saturate its entire structure. At once, your pancreas feels less congested and more invigorated to produce exactly the precise amount of insulin your body needs to take in sugar.

From the pancreas, the thick, golden liquid of sweetness coats all of your inner organs and then separates into two separate streams—one that travels down towards your toes, and one that travels upwards into your heart, arms, neck, and head. You are completely saturated with joy, with a lightness of being. Your body glistens with the liquid coursing through it. Your heart, bathed in sweet light, begins to radiate like the sun, only instead of light, it shines forth rays of sweetness and fulfillment. Your body has been reprogrammed to receive joy and pleasure in life. Whatever activities you do, you will find a way to squeeze the joy from them and savor it in your cells.

Now magnify your awareness to the level of the muscle and the liver. See them each glowing with delight, and along their perimeter, see all of their receptors for insulin perk up and become activated to receive exactly the amount of insulin they need to help their cells take up sugar. Inside all the individual cells of the liver and muscle are the tiny messengers responsible for the cell's processing of sugar; see them all come alive and be cleansed of any interference that may impede their activity. Every cell is completely free of debris, ready to receive the insulin message in the best way for you.

Any sugar that has accumulated in your bloodstream is automatically brought back into balance, as the appropriate amounts of sugar enter into these renewed cells and tissues. Your red blood cells are free of any sugar hanging on to them, and this freedom allows them to more effectively carry oxygen to your body tissues.

You feel energized. Your blood runs smoother through your blood vessels. Your internal organs become harmonized. Your mind is able to concentrate, your skin is clear, and you breathe in sweetness before opening your eyes to the world of joy before you!

Meditation: Meditate on the idea of sweetness. List all the ways you can make your life sweeter without indulging in external sources of sweeteners like sugar.

Hypertension (SEE BLOOD PRESSURE, HIGH)

Hyperthyroidism

Physical description: A condition of increased amounts of thyroid-hormone production by the thyroid gland, resulting in accelerated metabolism, weight loss without changes in food intake, rapid or irregular heartbeat, sweating, and nervousness.

Energy center(s): Solar plexus, throat

Nourishment: *Diet*—(1) Consume a whole-foods, predominantly plant-based diet that is higher in calories to compensate for increased metabolism; (2) Eat small, frequent meals throughout the day to keep energy levels stable; (3) Avoid dietary stimulants such as caffeine; (4) Reduce intake of iodized salt. *Supplements*—(1) Protein supplement (e.g., rice, whey) to replace protein loss from any muscle breakdown; (2) A high-quality multivitamin and mineral (containing vitamins A, C and E, as well as calcium); (3) L-carnitine to help improve symptoms.

Emotion(s): Fear, fight-or-flight feeling, anxiety, uncertainty

Limiting belief(s): I burn up my resources. I run from the rhythm of my inner self. There are no brakes. Run, run, run! There is no time to look within.

Power animal: Turtle

Flower essence(s): Clematis, Morning Glory, Yarrow

Affirmation(s): A waterfall of forgiveness, calmness, and peace flows from within. I honor my body's natural rhythm. I am in harmony with my inner and outer environments.

Visualization: Close your eyes and place two fingers gently at the base of your neck, where your thyroid gland is located. Envision your thyroid gland as a beautiful, aquamarine butterfly fluttering its wings rapidly without moving anywhere. The fast flutter represents the overactivity of your thyroid gland, a condition called hyperthyroidism. From this position, you view the butterfly with wonder, admiring its grace, and at the same time, you feel that you can help it to be free from its incessant pace and to instead move at a speed that is comfortable.

Open a simple dialogue with the butterfly, and ask it what it needs to be free. Then wait patiently for its response. Whatever word or words come forth from the butterfly, imagine you grant the butterfly its wish(es), and with each breath you take, you deliver to the butterfly what it needs, through the vehicle of your intention. The butterfly begins to absorb the intention and respond to you. The movement of its wings slows down slightly, and with each breath, it slows a little more, a little more, a little more, until the butterfly is sitting perfectly poised and still, in a place of harmony within its home of the base of your neck.

Your body and consciousness at this moment are in utter alignment with the butterfly's peace and calmness. Let yourself be nourished by this feeling by resting here for a couple of moments. Every cell in your body has slowed down its metabolic machinery to resonate to this peace.

And with this adjustment, you also begin to see tiny blue butterflies throughout the whole of your body—a parade of butterflies filling your being, imparting to you light, beauty, and balance. A turquoise glow emanates from your body. Using the current of your inhale, envision the trillions of butterflies flapping their wings to the flow of your breath. And with your exhale, they fly free, in a mist, around you, clearing your energy and liberating within you the expression of your true nature.

See the multitude of butterflies span the sky above you and then make their way into the distance and a field full of flowers. Each butterfly is infused with a new-found bliss. The butterfly of your thyroid comes back to its resting place, in the base of your neck. It now carries within its wings the quality of congruency and provides your thyroid gland with the right timing for the release of your thyroid hormones throughout the body.

Meditation: Enjoy a meditation of focusing on your rhythms. See if you can sit still and become aware of all of the movements and sounds you create, listening to the gurgling in your gut, the beat of your heart, and the whisper of your breath.

Hypotension (See Blood Pressure, Low)

Hypothyroidism

Physical description: A condition of low thyroid hormone production by the thyroid gland, resulting in fatigue, sensitivity to cold, weight gain, constipation, pale skin, muscle aches, brittle hair and nails, heavy menstrual periods, and depression.

Energy center(s): Solar plexus, throat

Nourishment: *Diet*—(1) Avoid raw foods that contain goitrogens (substances that interfere with the thyroid's iodine uptake). These foods include soybeans, peanuts, pine nuts, millet, and vegetables from the *Brassica* family, such as cabbage, mustard greens, turnips, radishes. Cooking these foods deactivates the goitrogens. (2) Eat a whole-foods, balanced diet consisting of primarily (organically grown) plant foods (fruits, legumes, vegetables, whole grains) and coldwater fish. *Supplements*—A high-quality multivitamin and mineral containing nutrients for the production and metabolism of thyroid hormone: vitamins A, B2, B3, B6, and C, and zinc, selenium, iron, and copper.

Emotion(s): Defeat, rejection

Limiting belief(s): I lack life. I feel trampled on, put upon. My true self lays dormant.

Power animal: Moose

Flower essence(s): Calendula, California Wild Rose, Larkspur

Affirmation(s): I move through life with ease and through expression. I am focused and determined to allow all my possibilities to blossom. I am genuinely warm towards myself and others. I take healthy risks. I infuse my inner authority with enthusiasm.

Visualization: Envision yourself covered with a sticky, slow-moving syrup that pours from the spigot of the base of your neck. With your inner eye, move through the internal landscape of your body, seeing how the syrup has permeated every cell, jamming up their machinery, making the parts stick together like glue. This syrup makes you feel lethargic and slows down all the functioning in your body. You feel like you live life in slow motion. The syrup can make you feel not only sluggish, but also weak and cold. In its presence, you feel that your brain is not as quick and able to remember as you'd like it to be, and your gut doesn't move materials through as fast as you'd like.

Set an intention to create movement throughout all layers of the body—physical, emotional, mental, spiritual, and any other layers you wish to address. Breathe in through the base of your neck, at your thyroid gland, and imagine your breath becomes a catalyst for alchemy, turning the cold metal of the spigot from which the syrup pours forth into shining, flexible gold and silver. See the gold and silver, the yang and yin, in perfect balance within your throat-chakra center. The spigot is bright and shiny, and the two colors swirl together.

The spigot transforms into a disc shape in the base of your throat. Like a wheel, it moves in a circular direction, casting off rays of gold and silver through your body, dissolving the sticky syrup that coats your inner being and prevents it from moving through life at an authentic pace. Each droplet of syrup is completely dried up and replaced with the fast-moving energy of an intertwining gold and silver light. You can actually see the inner landscape of your body now, without any veil of obstruction. All is clear and crystalline. Any buildup or decay has been transformed by the yang-yin disc of energy residing in your thyroid gland.

And you suddenly feel very alive, whole, and complete. You are imbued with a sense of purpose for living life to the fullest. You have the energy now to take on your passions, hobbies, and anything you wish. Let the yang-yin disc rotate at a speed that is appropriate for your body; this speed will determine the timing at which your body will disseminate thyroid hormones, in the perfect amount, to keep you healthy. Your body feels more light and less heavy and thick.

Throughout every layer of you, the gold-silver energy penetrates to release any stagnation, block, challenge, or negativity and open you up to the possibility of opportunity, flow, expression, and positivity. You allow your highest will to embrace this change.

And now, your thyroid gland functions optimally and smoothly. Verbally affirm, from the wellspring of your yang-yin energy in your throat, "I move through life with ease and expression." When you are ready, come back with your entire present self to the current moment.

Meditation: Focus your meditative energy on the radiance of the sunrise as it comes up on the horizon. Try this as often as you can. If you cannot access the sun rising, meditate on the color yellow. Build up warmth, heat, and activation energy in every cell of your body.

Impotence (SEE INFERTILITY)

Incontinence, Urinary

Physical description: The involuntary passage of urine from the urinary bladder due to problems with the muscles and nerves that hold or release urine.

Energy center(s): Root, sacral

Nourishment: *Diet*—(1) Avoid drinking excessive fluids or ingesting caffeine (tea, coffee, chocolate), alcohol, spicy foods, and citrus foods (including cranberry); (2) If you are overweight or obese, focus on reducing weight by eating a balanced, whole-foods diet abundant in low-glycemic-index fruits, vegetables, legumes, and whole grains.

Emotion(s): Fear, insecurity, helplessness, loss of integrity, feeling abandoned, feeling unsupported

Limiting belief(s): Fear moves through me and is beyond my control. I lack support and feel helpless in my situation. I look to others for validation. My boundaries are not defined.

Power animal: Fish

Flower essence(s): Heather, Yarrow

Affirmation(s): My emotions and creativity flow through me in the proper rhythm for my highest self. My inner self is supported with integrity and fulfillment.

Visualization: Imagine your body is like a house. Each compartment is its own room, and the different organ systems fulfill the various functions needed in the house. Our focus will be on the metaphorical plumbing system of the house—the kidneys, ureters, bladder, and urethra. The plumbing system in your body-house has a leak and needs repair. Envision yourself as the entire body, but also envision that a certain part of you, your consciousness, is a skilled plumber. You are invited to survey the situation due to your high level of expertise about this particular plumbing construct.

Use your special flashlight and equipment, and dive in deep into the depths of your body-house to find out why there is leaking inside the house. Move your hands and flashlight along the main water filters (known as the kidneys), the pipes (known as the ureters), the water tank for the house (known as the bladder), and finally, the outlet of water to the outside (known as the urethra). See if you can find where the moisture is coming from. What does your intuition say? What is overflowing and why? What has been held back to the point of pressure? When you find the place of sensitivity or place where there is a crack, use your special binding material to seal it up completely. Infuse strength into the plumbing system through your intention to do so.

Before you finish the job, run through all the plumbing apparatus a unique type of water—one that carries with it the energy of emotions and creativity. Run this water through the plumbing and allow for any stuck or clogged pipes to release old emotional debris or stagnant creativity. The pipes are now clear, strong, sealed, and durable.

Commend yourself for a job well done. And zoom yourself out of the plumber role slowly, coming back to your body image in its entirety, seeing it as a body rather than a house. Before progressing fully to the present moment, affirm to yourself, "My emotions and creativity flow through me in the proper rhythm for my highest self."

Meditation: List at least five ways that you can support your creativity. Try to implement one.

Indigestion

Physical description: Discomfort in the stomach area (upper abdomen) that manifests as bloating, belching, nausea, and/or fullness during and after a meal.

Energy center(s): Solar plexus, sacral, heart, throat

Nourishment: *Diet*—(1) Eat mindfully and slowly. Avoid talking while eating, or swallowing too much air by chewing with mouth open or gulping food. Be relaxed while eating; (2) Avoid drinking too much liquid with a meal, as stomach acid and digestive enzymes will become diluted, causing reduced digestion; (3) Work with a qualified healthcare professional to assess the presence of food allergies; (4) Emphasize fiber-rich foods, such as legumes, fruits, vegetables, and whole grains; (5) Avoid refined sugars, alcohol, spicy foods, dairy products, and fatty, processed foods; (6) Try eating monomeals, or single food items, limiting the complexity of multinutrient digestion. *Supplements*—(1) Digestive enzymes with a meal; (2) Take hydrochloric acid (as betaine HCl; use with caution or under the guidance of a healthcare professional) or apple cider vinegar with a meal if low stomach acid is the culprit; (3) A probiotic supplement; (4) A fiber supplement.

Emotion(s): Discomfort, uneasiness

Limiting belief(s): I am unable to digest my life events. I feel full and uncomfortable with what I am expected to take in. I refuse my personal power.

Power animal: Mouse

Flower essence(s): Dill, Indian Pink, Mountain Pride

Affirmation(s): I readily and quickly ingest, digest, and assimilate all form of nutrition—physical, emotional, mental, and spiritual. I sit comfortably in my radiant center. I digest my life fully and completely.

Visualization: Bring your awareness to your upper belly region by placing an open hand on your abdomen. Using your hand, see if you can feel or sense through the sense of touch what is occurring in this area of your body. Do you feel movement? Bloating? Pain? Do you feel acidity deep within? Whatever quality you pick up on through your hands or through any other senses, be sure to ask yourself why you have that quality. What message is your body trying to convey? Indigestion is a sign from your body that there may be things—whether they are situations, events, or dealings with others or even yourself—that you are trying to process, but it is not easy to run these things through yourself on a gut level, on a body level. There is resistance. See if you can take just a couple of moments to discern what those issues might be. What are you attempting to process that is causing you some discomfort? If nothing comes to you, stay with the discomfort and be in it as fully as you can. If you do get a "hit" as to what this is, stay with that specific event.

With your hands still on your belly, pull your breath down into your stomach, filling it with as much air as you can—almost like you were blowing air into a balloon. Let your hands rise with the filling of the belly. Invite the breath to circulate and stream through this area of discomfort, mixing with it, swirling around, getting the area moving with energy. And try this exercise again—breathing in to feel your belly rise into the palm of your hand, meeting your discomfort face to face, and then letting the belly sink down and into your body, like sinking into a pillow. The mere presence of the breath gives your stomach area some room to expand, so there is less constriction felt on a body level and more opening to the issues at hand. Use this openness to explore your body's ability to process and decipher information. What insight do you receive?

Breathe at your own pace for five to ten more breaths, or until you feel a sense of relaxation come through you like waves moving through the ocean. Unify all parts of yourself through your breath. As you are doing this, you may find that your abdominal discomfort or indigestion begins to dissipate, becoming lost to the currents of your breath.

Now form a vision of a porcelain crucible, or container for burning, in the area of your stomach. Make this container unique to you by including any design on the outside or inside. The container has a lid, which is attached and open. Bring in ideas, situations, foods, drinks, or interactions, letting them fall into the crucible, and then close the lid with your mind's eye. Burn the contents completely through with the element of digestive fire that resides in your gut. See your interaction as an offering to your spirit—a transformation of the outer world into a form that resonates with your inner world. Anytime you feel susceptible to indigestion or have digestive discomfort, uncover your inner crucible and use it to help you process, release, and transform whatever is causing you trouble.

When you are ready, let your hand fall away from your belly. Slowly return your awareness to the outer world, mentally affirming, "I can digest my life experience."

Meditation: One of the ways to better digest something is to break it up into smaller bites. How can you package your life events into more digestible bits? Meditate on this question and see what answers you receive.

Infertility

Physical description: The inability for a woman to become pregnant within one year of trying, and/or the inability for a pregnancy to be carried full term due to various causes, such as hormonal imbalances, decreased sperm motility (in men), and pelvic inflammatory disease.

Energy center(s): Root (men), sacral (women)

Nourishment: *Diet*—(1) Eat a low-glycemic-index, whole foods-based diet rich in fruits, vegetables, whole grains, nuts, and seeds; (2) Emphasize healthy oils, such as those rich in omega-3 fats, like flaxseed oil. *Supplements*—(1) Omega-3 fatty acid (fish or flax) supplement; (2) Acetyl-L-carnitine, L-carnitine, vitamin E, and coenzyme Q10 may be helpful for increasing sperm motility; (3) Chasteberry may assist with hormonal balance in women (check with your practitioner to discern whether your hormones need fine-tuning); (4) If blood sugar is imbalanced, focus on chromium, B-complex vitamin, green tea extract, and cinnamon.

Emotion(s): Inadequacy, insecurity, rejection

Limiting belief(s): I am empty and incapable. I reject my inner creativity. I box myself in with rigid thinking. I suppress my inner artist and child. I am in conflict with my sexuality.

Power animal: Rabbit

Flower essence(s): Evening Primrose, Indian Paintbrush, Iris, Sticky Monkeyflower, Zinnia

Affirmation(s): I am overflowing with abundance. My inner life presents me with a cornucopia of playfulness, sensuality, and creativity. I am a sensual artist. Life is magical, and I welcome the mystery. My inner child plays.

Visualization: Put on an imaginary pair of glasses that allows you to see your body in a new way: it enables you to only see the water parts of your body. When you look through the glasses, you see where your body contains water and where the water is flowing or stagnant. Observe that most of your body (between 60 and 80 percent) consists of water. See it throughout your body—swirling amongst all the cells, being filtered through your kidneys, moving through your gut, coursing through your bloodstream. Your body relies on the quantity of water it contains for functioning.

Scan your body and see if there are parts of your body where you need more water. If there are, then through your intention, add water in those places. Put your awareness into a small boat, so you can get immersed in the water in your body, and direct the boat to the lower part of your torso, to the area of your reproductive organs. Observe what the flow of water is like in this area. Is there movement? If so, what type? Is it chaotic or frenzied? Or is it still and quiet? Something in between? Establish harmonized flow within this part of you, allowing not only the water parts of you to better circulate, but also the blood and oxygen to come into this area more fully.

See the blue energy of water, the red energy of blood, and the white energy of oxygen spiraling together, weaving their way around your low-belly area and into your reproductive organs. Envision that your reproductive organs become more vital, vibrant, healthy, and welcoming of fertility. If you notice here any cobwebs of old relationship patterns, recognize what you learned from them, and then bless and release these outdated patterns from your life. If your reproductive organs are immobilized and barren because they are tightly bound and constricted by expectations, clip away all connections to these barriers. Let this area be as free and mobile as possible.

Fill this space not only with the blue, red, and white energy of vital substances, but also with a colorful, rainbowed energy of growth, new life, and creativity. Welcome your creative spirit. Allow it to dance and express! Let your low belly have a party!

And when you feel light and invigorated with the soul of play, take a deep breath into your belly, and with your breath, pull in the word *create.* See the energy of creativity swirl within your reproductive organs. Flush through your entire body a breath of creativity, balancing and restoring the creative potential of each cell in your being so it is optimal for you.

When you are ready, you can take off your special glasses, sit with a smile for at least a couple of seconds, and move forward into your day.

Meditation: For one full week, let go of any unnecessary structure, such as to-do lists, habits, or ruts that you have found yourself in (like eating the same thing every day for breakfast). Let yourself be free with your schedule and embrace your ability to be creative.

Inflammation

Physical description: Inflammation is a process that can occur in the body on two levels: the first is short-term inflammation that results from an acute injury (e.g., a wound, trauma), and the second is chronic, or longer term, inflammation, which underlies the origin of diseases such as cardiovascular disease. The hallmarks of inflammation are swelling, redness, and pain.

Energy center(s): Root

Nourishment: *Diet*—(1) Avoid fatty meats high in inflammatory fats (e.g., beef, chicken) and processed, nutrient-poor (junk) foods laden with trans fats (e.g., cakes, cookies, snack foods); (2) Incorporate anti-inflammatory foods, such as foods high in omega-3 fats (e.g., flaxseed, fish, nuts, seeds, leafy green vegetables); (3) Emphasize raw over cooked foods to reduce inflammatory compounds formed with high heat (called advanced glycation end products). *Supplements*—(1) Vitamin C plus bioflavonoids to aid in wound healing and connective tissue repair and to support immune system function; (2) Digestive enzymes in between meals to control inflammation; (3) Zinc to assist in immune system function; (4) Anti-inflammatory botanicals such as boswellia, ginger, and curcumin (from turmeric).

Emotion(s): Anger, rage, irritation, emotional pain

Limiting belief(s): No one notices my pain. I neglect my inner wounds. I ignore my internal signals. Life inflames me. Everything is an emergency.

Power animal: Salmon

Flower essence(s): Golden Ear Drops, Honeysuckle, Scarlet Monkeyflower

Affirmation(s): I pay attention. I am calm and cool. My needs are met. I am listened to, and I listen to others.

Visualization: Take a generous, deep breath in, and as your breath travels inward, open your mind's eye to view your inner landscape. As you go within, you begin to see parts of you that are on fire, whether blazing or smoldering. Scan your entire body for these fires. There may be some parts in your body where fires are just beginning or matches are being ignited. You will quickly be able to identify these areas, as these are the parts of your body that are inflamed—red, swollen, and in pain.

Now imagine you have available a calm, cool, aquamarine energy from the depths of the sea. Step back out of your body, and with a hose that you can easily modify the size of, spray your entire body with this cool, bluish energy, starting at the top of your head and working your way downward. Allow the droplets to form a fine mist that coats all of your organs and tissues and even drizzles down into your cells. As your body becomes saturated with this mist, you feel an overall cooling sensation in your body. Parts of you that were red and in pain are becoming normal and even healthier than they've ever been.

Now use the hose to drench other fiery places with this cooling, anti-inflammatory water energy. Spend a couple of seconds on every place, so all large fires are put out, all smoldering ceases, and any hint of a match to be lighted is squelched. Let the water pool in these places. Feel the soothing, relaxed, flowing feeling spread within you like an ocean wave. You go with the flow of this peace, letting go of any stress, preoccupation, or inflammation about something in your life.

And now that you feel stronger and relieved of inflammation, let's bolster your cells with happiness. Have the energy of happiness and acceptance travel to all of the receptors on your cells' surfaces throughout your entire body, making them full of bliss. Let the bliss program your DNA, so you turn on only genes that will create contentment, beauty, and health. Take some time to ensure that all your cells receive this message, and when you are ready, come back to the present moment, bathed in a sea of cool, relaxed bliss.

Meditation: Focus your attention on a single flame from a candle. See the flame as a representative of the inflammation that burns within your body. Sit with the flame in peace, finding stillness in its intensity. Use the flame to dialogue with your own inner inflammation. At the end of the meditation, blow out the candle, setting a final intention to quell your inner heat to a level that is conducive to your health and healing.

Insomnia

Physical description: Sleep disturbance involving the inability to fall asleep, remain asleep, and get a good quality and quantity of sleep.

Energy center(s): Third eye

Nourishment: *Diet*—(1) Avoid or limit stimulating foods, such as caffeine, tobacco, cheese, chocolate, tomatoes, alcohol, and high-sugar foods, especially before bedtime; (2) Eat foods high in tryptophan, such as turkey, bananas, almond butter, or yogurt, close to bedtime; (3) Work with a qualified healthcare professional to identify food allergies; (4) Eat small, frequent meals throughout the day to prevent blood sugar imbalances. *Supplements*—(1) B-complex vitamin to encourage stress reduction and balanced metabolism and neurotransmitter levels; (2) A mineral supplement containing calcium and magnesium for muscle relaxation; (3) 5-hydroxytryptophan (5-HTP) to assist with neurotransmitter (serotonin) balance; (4) Melatonin if body levels are low; (5) Botanicals with sedative properties, such as passionflower, hops, and valerian.

Emotion(s): Worry, feeling overwhelmed, preoccupation

Limiting belief(s): I am overwhelmed. There is no time to take care of what needs tending to. My mind is cluttered and busy. I refuse to look at the messages in my dreams.

Power animal: Bear

Flower essence(s): Cherry Plum, Lavender, Mimulus, White Chestnut

Affirmation(s): I can rest when needed. I trust that everything will be taken care of in due time. I release chaos from my mind. My brain and nervous system are perfectly harmonized. I am in tune with the powerful information revealed to me in my dreams.

Visualization: Close your eyes and take a gentle breath in and a soft exhale out. Allow your internal gaze to drift upwards towards the middle of your forehead. Breathe into this space and see here a bright, violet star. This star lives within this sacred, intuitive space, acting as your internal guide and messenger. As you breathe into this brilliant star, it becomes even brighter and more sparkling. It is fed by your breath and focus. Its luminescence fills your head, casting out any old thoughts from the past that have collected in your mind like piles of trash. These thoughts no longer serve you, and so you release them to the star. Its healing light balances all neural circuitry.

Instead of the nerves firing and neurotransmitters being congested like rush-hour traffic, they are now streamlined and flowing at a pace that is perfect for you. Your thoughts become quieter, not as noisy and disruptive. In fact, they are so subdued and controlled that you can now parcel away your thoughts, like putting away books on a library shelf. With the help of the violet starlight, your mind becomes tidy and full of order. It becomes clean and shiny. Any residual worry has been transformed to trust because everything is in its place. You can access any thoughts you need upon your own wish to do so. However, they will no longer be disorganized.

Your mind is fed by this star, and you are able to call upon it for nourishment whenever you feel you need to release the chaos from your mind. The star is there to guide and direct your thoughts back into place. Breathing gently while focusing on the star, let the light of the star intensify, enabling one of its penetrating rays to move down from your head to the middle of your body. Allow the starlight to permeate your belly, like a laser, to release any held stress or tension. Guide the laser to where you need it most, moving it through the heat of your stomach area, cutting through any anger in your liver, dissolving unfelt emotions in your intestines. Move all pain and stress through the body into the violet starlight, letting them dissolve and wither away.

Fill this part of you, instead, with a sense of balance. Visualize this area of your body like a calm body of water. Only you have the ability to make the water ripple or create waves. Right now, you feel the peace of the water. You will always remember how to connect with this peacefulness.

Move the violet starlight into your legs and feet, removing any blocks to trust in your life. Make sure to bask your knees in this light so they have the ability to move you forwards and backwards when you need them to. Let any distrust or mistrust dissolve and run through the soles of your feet. Replace the lack of trust with pillars of loving protection and security. Allow your legs and feet to be warm with the trust of knowing that all happens perfectly, in its own time.

From here, guide the starlight back up to your head and run it through your body seven more times to ensure that you are balanced and full of a wellspring of calm. See the violet star in your mind's eye once again, letting it blanket you with the ability to rest and sleep soundly. With your permission, the star will lead you safely into the dream world to explore and release your earthly preoccupations. Let go, let go, let go.

Meditation: Lie in bed as if you were ready to go to sleep. Your arms are at your sides, and your head rests comfortably on a pillow. Starting at your feet, tense your feet, ankles, and up into your legs, buttocks— your entire body all the way up to your face. Feel the tension you have gathered in your body surfacing. Let it all come to the top. Now imagine an ocean wave washing over you, starting at your feet and progressing to your head. Feel the tension release, like an ocean wave moving through you. Practice this progressive relaxation in silence and with an empty mind until you feel soft, supple, and unstressed.

Interstitial Cystitis (SEE URINARY TRACT INFECTION)

Irritable Bowel Syndrome (IBS)

Physical description: A common gastrointestinal disorder that involves abdominal pain and discomfort and alternating patterns of defecation (i.e., constipation and diarrhea), often coinciding with periods of stress and anxiety.

Energy center(s): Sacral, solar plexus

Nourishment: *Diet*—(1) Avoid or limit caffeine, dairy products (except small amounts of plain, unsweetened yogurt, if it can be tolerated), alcohol, gluten-containing grains (barley, rye, wheat, spelt, oat), and refined sugars; (2) Emphasize high-fiber fruits and vegetables; (3) Work with a qualified healthcare professional to identify food allergies. *Supplements*—(1) Probiotics *(Lactobacillus acidophilus, Bifidobacterium bifidum)*; (2) Enteric-coated peppermint oil.

Emotion(s): Apprehension, self-doubt, feeling overwhelmed, irritation

Limiting belief(s): People irritate me. I am overwhelmed. Emotions sit in a ball in my belly. No one understands all that I have to process. I am stuck and stagnant in my emotions.

Power animal: Whale

Flower essence(s): Aspen, Chamomile, Dill, Filaree, Sagebrush

Affirmation(s): I am receptive and creative. I allow a flow of energy to clear all stagnation from my gut and to introduce harmony and healing. I welcome change. I flow with all of life. I invite my emotions to express their full selves without fear or worry. I am dynamic.

Visualization: Place both hands on your low belly and feel the rise and fall of your deep belly breaths. See your belly like the ocean. Notice how it rises gently on the inhale, filling with peace and calm, allowing a warm, liquid sensation to flow throughout your entire being. First it flows to the upper parts of your body—to your upper torso and neck, out your head, and then down your shoulders, moving out of your fingertips. And then the warmth extends to your lower body—moving to your hips, running down your thighs, spiraling around your knees, and flowing into your feet until it can exit through your toes. You have become the ocean, and your belly is the center of your universe in this moment. You feel secure and nourished by these beautiful glistening waters.

Sometimes the waves feel strong and forceful. With a supportive inhale, you meet those waves with your breath and carry them through your body and out your fingertips and toes. And in a moment, you feel at rest.

Put all of your attention into your belly region. Infuse honor and gratitude into your belly, thanking it for all of its many functions, like transforming information from the outside into internal information and filtering through that which you need. Affirm to your gut that you willingly receive what it takes in, as you trust that it provides only that for your highest self. It removes all that you do not need or that serves you incorrectly. Look at your belly with wonder for its ability to transmit information to you—emotions, creativity, sensuality. It provides you with many gifts and offerings so you can create a healing path.

See any unexpressed emotions swirling within your belly and allow them to dance and spiral together. Release them into the space around you, giving them space to express themselves. Observe their movement. See if they have messages for you. Tell yourself that you will receive and remember all of their messages and use this information for healing.

Buried in the depth of your low abdomen you find a treasure chest— an ancient one, like you might find in the bowels of the ocean.

And here is your own treasure chest in the depth of your universal water. It is the chest of creativity. The moment you open it, you will find your gifts, talents, skills, and creativity, all ready to greet you. Now open the treasure chest slowly and examine its contents. What do you find? How do you respond to its contents? For every object, look at it carefully, with a loving gaze, and breathe into it your heartfelt gratitude. Listen to the guidance of each one. Make a mental note of all these gifts of creativity and know that in your daily living you will embrace each of them individually, like children, and nourish their growth in your own unique ways.

Now close the chest of creativity and put it back into your belly, in a place that you can easily find it. Bow to all of your emotions, honoring them for their information. Take a nice, deep inhale, again feeling your hands on your belly. See a swirl of bright red-orange energy closing this space, like a sunset.

Meditation: Lie down or sit comfortably and give yourself a gentle, meditative belly massage, moving clockwise from your lower right abdomen up the right side, over the expanse of the torso, under the diaphragm, and down the left side. After a couple of times, rest your hands, one on top of the other, in the center of your belly region and focus on your breath for the remainder of the meditation.

Itching

Physical description: An irritation in the skin that causes one to scratch the area; commonly seen as a symptom of allergies, eczema, dry skin, insect bites/stings, parasitic infection, and stress, and associated with use of certain medications.

Energy center(s): Root, crown

Nourishment: *Diet*—(1) Work with a qualified healthcare professional to assess whether food allergies are present; (2) Reduce refined carbohydrates and yeast-containing foods, like bread, in case of *Candida albicans* overgrowth; (3) Eat a whole-foods, hypoallergenic diet consisting primarily of plant foods. Eliminate or reduce dairy products, meats, shellfish, citrus foods, and gluten-containing grains. *Supplements*—(1) Detoxifying herbs to support liver function, such as silymarin and green tea extract; (2) Probiotic supplement.

Emotion(s): Irritation, feeling overwhelmed

Limiting belief(s): I am itching to get out of here. Something under the surface of a particular situation is irritating to me. I don't feel comfortable in my skin.

Power animal: Snake

Flower essence(s): Agrimony, Chrysanthemum, Rosemary

Affirmation(s): I am liberated from any limiting, irritating situation. I find myself enveloped in calm and comfort. Deep within every encounter lies soulful wisdom. My true self surfaces in the form of silky skin.

Visualization: Close your eyes; relax fully. Let your hand receive a magical, energized, soft-bristled brush. Notice that when you rub your other hand on the brush, it feels soft, yet stimulating.

Breathe in and set an intention for working with your skin. Ask your skin to prepare to release that which is itching it. Move the brush over the landscape of your skin, starting with the top of your left shoulder and gliding it down both sides of your arm, the upper side and then the lower side. Feel your skin letting go of all its troubles, worries, concerns, and unexpressed emotions. Then brush your armpit area to invigorate the lymph nodes, continuing down the side body and then making your way up to the top of your chest. Work your way down with the brush in a slow, rhythmic, intentional way. As best you can, reach over your left shoulder to brush away anything that has been burdensome or tiring, and then scoop your right hand with the brush underneath your left arm to get at your middle and low back. Bring to the surface any lack of support you feel and any feelings that you have around not being supported in your life. Brush those away.

Move the brush down your left leg, including your thigh, knee, and calf and even the top of your left foot. Expel any and all impediments that are related to your past and that have made their way under your skin. Brush your inner and outer left leg, and feel the stretch of circulation that is being stimulated to move things through. And now slowly brush the back of your left leg from top to bottom, starting at your left buttock and ending at your left ankle.

Shake out the brush; let everything it has collected, which serves you incorrectly, be released into the ground beneath you. Set an intention for the transformation of all that you have released.

And now, putting the brush in your left hand, start at your right shoulder and work your way down your right arm, on the top and under it, allowing any stigmas or limiting beliefs about being open to receiving from others to fall away, completely and fully. Move the brush down the right side of your chest in short, rhythmic strokes, helping to shed anything that blocks your heart, lungs, or digestive tract. Ensure that you take a few seconds to wipe your upper right back with the brush, removing any resentment, and your middle to lower right back to dispel any issues related to money or stress that are detrimental to you at this time.

Once you feel that you have been thorough enough, trace the brush down your right leg, including your thigh, knee, shin, and top of the foot. Shake the brush out, releasing any accumulated stuck energy or preoccupations about the future. Take some time to brush your back right leg, starting with your buttock and moving slowly down to your ankle. Again, shake out the brush like a rattle, letting any energetic debris fall away from you and be absorbed by the earth.

Put the brush down and use both of your hands to comb through your hair, over your scalp. Move your fingers over your face, letting go of any mind patterns that are self-defeating, and invigorating your brain and face with a whole new approach to life that serves you and others in the best way.

Once you are done brushing your skin, stand tall, with your arms at either side, and imagine you are being coated with a honeylike, slippery liquid that covers you from top to bottom—every inch of you, every crack and crevice. It provides an energetic blanket of peace and acceptance, preventing you from itching and events and people from getting under your skin. With this coating, which is invisible to others, but apparent to you, you feel safe and protected. Your boundaries have been reset, and your skin glows with confidence and strength!

Meditation: If you are feeling itchy, zoom into one itch in particular and ask it, "What are you itching me to pay attention to?" Let yourself be in the moment fully and completely and wait for it to respond. Journal what you feel/sense/hear/intuit.

Jaundice (SEE LIVER PROBLEMS)

Jaw Tightness (Temporomandibular Joint, or TMJ)

Physical description: The jaw clenches periodically throughout the day and night, causing muscle tightness and soreness in the mouth, jaw, neck area.

Energy center(s): Throat

Nourishment: *Diet*—(1) Avoid foods that cause stress and inflammation in the body: refined sugar and flour, soft drinks, fast foods, baked goods, caffeine; (2) Eat a healthy diet consisting of vegetables, whole grains, legumes, and cold-water fish. *Supplements*—(1) Glucosamine sulfate to support the integrity of the jaw structure; (2) Vitamin C and B-complex vitamins (particularly pantothenic acid, or vitamin B5) to help the body combat stress.

Emotion(s): Anger, rage, frustration

Limiting belief(s): I am too angry to speak. My authentic voice is trapped within me.

Power animal: Eagle

Flower essence(s): Agrimony, Cosmos, Red Clover, Scarlet Monkey-flower, Snapdragon

Affirmation(s): I speak my truth freely. My voice is powerful and needs to be heard. What I have to say is valuable. My words are crafted with honesty, integrity, and truth.

Visualization: Open your mouth slightly and close your eyes. Breathe deeply, using your mouth rather than your nose. Let your breath expand your jaw just a little until you feel that your jaw is relaxed. As it becomes more relaxed, you start to release pressure, like a balloon that is deflating. Your jaw becomes heavy, as though sandbags were attached to all four corners underneath its structure. And as your mouth begins to soften, pay attention to any soreness or tenderness within, and send patches of loving kindness to these areas.

Now visualize that you are presented with a blue and green lozenge. Put the lozenge on your tongue and invite it to dissolve very gradually. With the melting of the lozenge, the inside of your mouth, including your gums, teeth, upper palate, tongue, and sides of your mouth become coated with relaxation. You may even see images or text floating from your mouth as you let go of that which holds you back. The cooling essence of the lozenge begins to permeate your jaw deeper and deeper, sinking into the bony structure, dampening any inflammation. As it does so, your mind wanders its way to any past or recent situations where you expressed words, beliefs, or opinions that may have been considered inflammatory by others. Let those events unwind themselves from the matrix of your jaw. You can let go of them, like letting a kite travel into the summer sky. You watch them become smaller and smaller, transforming into a speck in the sky and then disappearing completely. How liberated you feel from this release!

And now, go even deeper into your mouth cavity, searching it as if it were a dark cave. Look for words, messages, opinions, beliefs that you *wish* you had expressed at one time, but never did because of fear or the potential of retaliation. When we box up our expressions, they turn inward and create pain within our body. And so they must be let go in some form. Visualize those intentions and expressions freeing themselves, like bats flying through the cave of your mouth and out into the blinding sunshine. Now is your opportunity to shine light on all that has been hidden and festering, especially any tension or anger.

With your jaw now fully expanded, relaxed, and empty of anything said or unsaid that has held you back, drink from a glass containing the liquid light of truth. With each sip, enjoy its soft radiance swirling in the region of your mouth. See the liquid light saturate all structures in your mouth and seep down into your jaw, crystallizing its essence there and leaving no room for anger, fear, jealousy, ego, rage, or resentment. Your mouth feels fluid and light, and it is programmed with a new template—that all words and speech created and traveling from it are encased in the brilliance of the liquid light of truth.

Bring your focus back to your breath, breathing in through your mouth. Slowly close your mouth and open your eyes. Mentally affirm, "I speak my truth."

Meditation: Lightly massage your jaws with your fingertips. And as you do so, meditate on what words are stored within the confines of your jaws. What have you wanted to say? Capture the words and phrases in your journal. Think of creative ways in which you can express these words in the next week (e.g., poetry, collage, song, dialogue with a friend, essay).

Kidney Stones

Physical description: Hard mineral crystal deposits on the inner surface of the kidney(s) that cause extreme pain when passing into the bladder.

Energy center(s): Root, sacral

Nourishment: *Diet*—(1) Eat a diet of low-glycemic-index and high fiber foods—fruits, vegetables, and whole grains; (2) Reduce your intake of refined sugar, alcohol, salt, and animal products (especially organ meats, shellfish, and high-calcium dairy foods); (3) Eat magnesium-rich foods like whole grains (e.g., brown rice, barley, buckwheat, rye), nuts (e.g., cashew, peanuts), seeds (e.g., sesame seeds), and potatoes; (4) Emphasize green, leafy vegetables, which are high in vitamin K, a stone inhibitor; (5) Drink adequate water throughout the day to dilute the urine; (6) If stones are comprised of oxalate, limit oxalate-containing foods, like black tea, cocoa, spinach, nuts, parsley, vegetables in the cabbage family, and cranberries. *Supplements*—If stones contain calcium: (1) B-complex vitamins; (2) Vitamin K; (3) Magnesium. If stones contain uric acid: Folic acid.

Emotion(s): Rigidity, bitterness, anger, strife

Limiting belief(s): I resist flowing in the stream of life events. My anger overwhelms my ability to move forward with ease and without pain. I am bitter about letting go.

Power animal: Fish

Flower essence(s): Angel's Trumpet, Black-eyed Susan, Dogwood, Honeysuckle, Walnut

Affirmation(s): A seamless river of life-force energy flows through me, removing that which needs clearing, and revitalizing that which nourishes me. I dance with life, and life dances with me. I forgive.

Visualization: Close your eyes, rub your hands together quickly until you feel some warmth rise in your palms, and place them in the area of your kidneys—on your middle- to lower-back area at the outer ends. Pour your healing, pooled life force into this area of your body. Sit with this feeling for a couple of seconds. Continue to breathe with awareness, bringing each breath to the site of the kidneys. With each breath, they become more and more alive and vibrant in your body.

At any point during this visualization, you can let your hands go, allowing them to dangle by your sides.

With each long-lasting, meaningful moment, become aware that each of your kidneys holds the essence of your life. They are treasure chests for your vitality and longevity and the source of life-force energy. By strengthening your kidneys, you will increase your stamina and energy level.

Visualize that, with each breath, you drift down to the bottom of a vast sea until your finally arrive at the bottom to find these two gem-laden chests, which are your kidneys. Take the chest on your left and open it. What do you find here? Do you see any objects, and, if so, what significance do these objects have for you? What do your findings say about your feminine side and your lineage of female ancestors that goes back endlessly to the beginning of time? Enjoy fishing around in this voluminous container. Note if anything you find carries strong emotions, like anger or sadness, and if so, observe, acknowledge, give thanks, and then let it drift away in the ocean currents rather than be sealed up in this box containing your precious life energy.

When you feel ready, swim over to the treasure chest on your right. Compare its appearance with that of the chest on the left. And in perfect time, observe its contents, just like you did with the other chest. What types of objects do you find, and what is your reaction to them? Let the objects float out of the chest so you can behold them at all levels and interact with them if needed. Are there any messages for your masculine nature in this box? How do you feel this treasure chest and its contents connect you to your lineage of male ancestors going back to the beginning of time? Sink into these moments fully and completely. Be ready to release any emotional charges that you may have attached to any of the stored items. Let those float away into the depths of the ocean.

And now, with your mind's eye, which has amazing potential to transform anything it chooses, adjust the boxes to look exactly how you want them to. Redesign and beautify them to suit the essence of who you are—your highest self. With your breath as a means of support, let the treasure chests move upwards towards the ocean surface.

When the treasure chests reach the surface, they are magically transported onto a boat. You climb onto the deck of the boat, looking down at the boxes. Take both of your hands once again and rub them together quickly to generate a generous cloud of life-force energy. Point your left hand in the direction of your left treasure chest and your right hand in that of the right treasure chest. Feel your energy extending to your treasures, your kidneys. Visualize that energy streaming out of you and into the two boxes. And at the same time, see liquid vibrance flowing from the treasure chests into your hands.

After taking in this vibrant energy, place your hands on your actual kidneys once again and let the liquid energy saturate through to your kidneys. See them becoming renewed, clear, vital, and able to do their tasks of filtering toxins through the fluid portion of your body. Mentally affirm, "A seamless river of life-force energy flows through me, removing that which needs clearing, and revitalizing that which nourishes me."

Meditation: Meditate on your blocks of bitterness and anger that prevent you from forgiving and moving on. Write a letter about your feelings, addressing it to the person on whom the anger or bitterness centers, but do not send the letter.

Knee Pain

Physical description: Pain felt in the knee region due to swelling and inflammation from acute injury, arthritis, gout, or infection.

Energy center(s): Root

Nourishment: *Diet*—Emphasize anti-inflammatory foods (fruits, vegetables, fish, legumes, whole grains) in place of inflammatory, meat-based foods. *Supplements*—(1) Digestive enzymes in between meals; (2) Joint-supporting nutrients, such as glucosamine and chondroitin; (3) Anti-inflammatory botanicals, like boswellia, ginger, curcumin, and bioflavonoids (e.g., quercetin).

Emotion(s): Feeling stuck (in the past or future), fear, reluctance

Limiting belief(s): I cannot go further. I am stuck in the pain of the past. Fear makes me unwilling to look at the future. I am held back and stuck.

Power animal: Dragonfly

Flower essence(s): Arnica (if injury present), Blackberry, Dogwood

Affirmation(s): I move forward effortlessly and gracefully. I am filled with hope in place of fear. I glide through life's challenges. I continually increase my awareness as I am moving through the world.

Visualization: Place your hands on your knees—the left hand on the left knee and the right hand on the right knee. Take a gentle breath in, followed by a slow exhale.

Put your attention into your left knee first. On your next inhale, imagine your leg as a hollow tube. See your left knee as a valve that can be opened and released, much like a kitchen faucet can. With your mind's eye, slowly open the valve in your left knee, allowing whatever needs to pour through from your past to move through the hollow tube of your leg, exit through the sole of your foot, and travel into the ground beneath you. See past wounds, harbored memories, sticky situations of old and watch them unglue themselves from the left knee. You can control the flow of these collected tokens of the past by simply turning up or down the release valve of this knee. Like molasses, these past residues make their way through your leg and out your foot. The loving earth absorbs the hurts, resentments, and anger left behind in your body and transforms them into tools that will nourish and replenish you at this time. Your left foot drinks back in the transformed energy, which is now fast moving rather than like the slow, dripping molasses. This energy moves up into your leg and finally to your knee. Your left knee basks in the glow of this newfound energy. It feels new and cleansed of all debris from the past. It is illuminated with the green energy that comes from stepping into a new realm that is clear and welcoming of change.

From here, shift your awareness to your right knee. Breathe into this knee, causing the energy contained within it to settle down. The flurry inside your right knee dissipates. You pick up pieces of what has settled in the knee, noticing all the concerns of the future: concerns about money, shelter, relationships, family matters. All the "what ifs" of your life have anchored themselves in the terrain of your right knee, causing you to feel their pain penetrating your knee. Like stakes pinning something to the ground, they prevent you from truly moving forward at a pace that is best for you. One by one, you remove all the worry and what-if stakes that have pierced your right knee. Each one is removed with love and compassion and set aside. Put all the pieces of what no longer serves you into a large garbage can. And, in an instant, imagine all of those useless worries being burned to ashes. As they burn away, the warmth and support you need at your core is delivered to your right knee. At the end of their burning, your knee is filled with the hope and possibility of the present moment. Your preoccupation with the future has evaporated, liberating your true nature, which is able to take things as they come, to walk in a comfortable stride through life.

Now, placing your focus into both your knees, imagine a figure eight, or the symbol of infinity, spiraling back and forth over both knees to bring them into unison. The past and future of your life walk together in harmony, moving you fully and gracefully into the present moment. You welcome the change and move on.

Meditation: In a quiet setting, contemplate on that which holds you back in the past or keeps you fixated on the future. See if you can find all parts of yourself collected in the present moment.

Left-Side-of-Body Complaints

Physical description: The left side of the body corresponds to the feminine (yin) part of our nature—that which is creative, emotional, introspective, and dynamic. A greater proportion of symptoms on the left side of the body would indicate that there is an imbalance in that quality of one's life.

Energy center(s): Sacral, heart, third eye

Nourishment: Fat is the nutrient with the most feminine resonance, as it is helps the body to communicate to itself through the flow of substances in and out of the cells. If you are deficient in feminine energy, eating more liquid, vegetable-based fats (e.g., oils from olives, flaxseed, walnuts, and sesame seeds) may be harmonizing. Conversely, if there is too much feminine nature, reducing fat may be of benefit.

Emotion(s): Aggression (if feminine energy is deficient) or insecurity (if feminine energy is excessive)

Limiting belief(s): Challenges with nurturing and mother figures. *If feminine energy is deficient*: I give up my creativity and ability to nourish my inner, emotional realm. *If feminine energy is excessive*: I overnurture others and neglect myself.

Power animal: Heron

Flower essence(s): Alpine Lily, Calendula (if deficient), Evening Primrose, Fuchsia (if deficient), Indian Paintbrush (if deficient), Mariposa Lily

Affirmation(s): The feminine part of my nature is balanced. I am in harmony. The yin and yang within me are in equal measure. I am yielding and nurturing with myself and others. I let my creative, emotive self swirl and spiral within and outside of me.

Visualization: Envision an invisible, electric blue line that divides the left and right sides of your body. Use this marker as a way to focus your attention on the left side of you—your feminine, healing side. This is the part of you that receives from and is receptive to people, as well as to your own creativity and inner voice. It is the deep-knowledge part of you. See the left side as the yin and the right side as the yang of your being; your left side is colored white, and your right side is colored black.

Focus now on the yin side of you. Engage your yin in a dialogue with the following questions: How do I receive? Am I open to my inner voice? Do I tap into my wellspring of creativity? How do I access the inner healer in me for myself and for others? Do I listen, reflect, and contemplate my actions, or do I simply act aggressively? See what part of you enters into this dialogue. What answers do you *receive?*

The more you are able to mine the depth of your left side, the more it begins to morph from being the white of yin into an array of colors—red, orange, yellow, green, blue, violet. They begin to dance, flower, bloom, and spiral through the left side of your body, from head to toe. They are like the iridescent colors within oil—all working together, yet separate—and this spectrum permeates all parts of the left side of your body that need healing and receptivity. After the color absorbs into the left side, what is left is an array of water droplets, running together, pooling, collecting, and moving with the rhythm of your healing, feminine self, unlocking any creative impulses you may have. Your entire left side becomes like the ocean. Its watery depths move to the surface so you can dive deeper into your self. It will swirl and create activity with your intention to do so, and it will be calm and quiet with your intention to be still and receive.

Now that you have cultivated a sense of flow and movement within your left side, bring it together with the right side of you—the yang, active part of your nature. The black of the yang converts into flames of action. Become aware once again of the invisible, electric blue line that divides your left and right sides. Take a small circle of the water energy of your left side and plant it into your right side. Then take a small circle of the fire energy of your right side and secure it safely into your left side. Your being is balanced, and your dual natures are harmonized.

Meditation: Engage your creative, healer nature in meditative writing. Let this part of you write without being controlled or censored, for at least three minutes per day.

Liver Problems

Physical description: The liver is a key organ for the digestion, assimilation, and metabolic regulation of nutrients, along with the release of toxins from the body. Symptoms of liver problems (such as hepatitis, bile-duct obstruction, fatty liver, and cirrhosis) include yellowish skin and eyes, abdominal pain, swelling, itchy skin, fatigue, nausea, loss of appetite, and changes in color of urine and/or stool.

Energy center(s): Solar plexus

Nourishment: *Diet*—(1) Avoid alcohol, fatty animal-based products, refined carbohydrates, and saturated and trans fats; (2) Eat primarily plant-based, high-fiber foods: brown rice; steamed or raw cruciferous vegetables, like broccoli, brussels sprouts, and cabbage; high-sulfur foods, such as garlic, onions, and eggs; legumes; and pears and apples. *Supplements*—(1) A high-potency multivitamin and mineral without iron; (2) Vitamin C; (3) Selenium; (4) N-acetylcysteine; (5) Alpha lipoic acid; (6) Liver-protective botanicals, such as silymarin (milk thistle), turmeric, and licorice.

Emotion(s): Anger, despair, hopelessness, depression

Limiting belief(s): Anger accumulates within me. My body cannot process the toxins of life. I am stagnant and suffering in a mire of hopelessness. My body and spirit are not integrated.

Power animal: Bull

Flower essence(s): Angelica, Blackberry, Lotus, Mallow, Scarlet Monkeyflower

Affirmation(s): Anger is a natural catalyst, and I use it to propel me into action. I move forward with my will. I free my body of toxins. My liver is renewed and refreshed. My body and spirit are perfectly aligned.

Visualization: It is autumn, and you are standing at the edge of a field, looking into a vast expanse. You are wearing clothes that are loose and that hang on you comfortably, and you stand in a comfortable warrior stance—both feet planted on the ground, knees slightly bent. Your eyes look forward from under heavy eyelids.

In this moment, the energy of your liver moves from the inside to the outside, and it blankets your entire body. As you peer out into the distance, a current of autumnal air swirls around your feet, and with increasing speed, it funnels up your entire body—up your legs; into your torso, especially around the space where your liver resides (your upper right side); and then up into your lungs and heart. Finally, it whirls on through your neck and head and then flows out to rejoin the larger current of air from which it came. In its active, healthy state, the liver enjoys movement and activity and welcomes any catalysts to keep it in motion. The flow of air has helped to get inside your deeper layers to dislodge any stagnation, blocks, challenges, old negative patterns, and beliefs. It has created motion on very deep levels and induced stirrings in the liver, the seat of much stagnation.

And now see around you the visual portrayal of what situations or people you have allowed to block you. See them clearly, and with a fresh current of air, allow them to be swept away. Invite all the fallen leaves from the trees in the surrounding field to fly around you and carry them away, each leaf carrying away an impediment to your progress. If you feel any anger rising within you, take a look at it closely, as if you were observing it rather than feeling it. Note what you see. Give thanks to your anger, as it is a call to action, to your deepest path. And once this anger has expressed itself, let its remnants be swept away by the leaves, carried up into the bare tree branches.

Hear distant flute music floating through the breeze, dispersing and diffusing negativity and making way for the circulation of vitality in the air. Let yourself fall into the comfort of your breath, like a baby relaxing into its mother's arms. You enrobe yourself in a sense of trust and lightness, harmony restored.

See the naked tree branches starting to bud with new beginnings. The energy of the greenery and growth permeates your body, particularly the layer of your liver, which is at the forefront. Like seedlings, your body and spirit are receptive to that which nourishes them. You become a vibrant form of life, and all the structures around you in your life, which are like the supporting trees in the background, are thriving with energy to provide you with sustenance.

Transitioning from autumn into the newness of spring, you rebirth yourself to healthy movement and action in your life. Your liver is renewed and refreshed.

Meditation: When you feel anger, close your eyes and see it moving you in a particular direction. Follow it and see where it goes.

Memory Loss

Physical description: The state of being forgetful or consistently being unable to recall past events. May be permanent or temporary and have a sudden or gradual onset.

Energy center(s): Third eye

Nourishment: *Diet*—(1) Eat a low-glycemic-index, Mediterranean-style, plant-based diet full of whole grains, legumes, vegetables, and oils; (2) Eat anti-inflammatory foods, such as cold-water fish; all berries (strawberries, blueberries); green, leafy vegetables; nuts, olive and flaxseed oils; seeds; and spices such as turmeric and cinnamon; (3) Avoid refined carbohydrates. *Supplements*—(1) A high-quality, high-potency multivitamin and mineral; (2) Omega-3 (from flax or fish oil) supplement for reducing inflammation; (3) Ginkgo biloba, huperzine A, and phosphatidylserine are other supplements to consider.

Emotion(s): Denial, despair, feeling overwhelmed

Limiting belief(s): I am losing my mind. I refuse to accept aging. I reject my past.

Power animal: Elephant

Flower essence(s): Cerato, Indian Pink, Penstemon

Affirmation(s): I cherish my internal wisdom. I remember everything I choose to. I am centered within my mind. I am endowed with clarity, perspective, and insight.

Visualization: Close the curtains of your eyelids and let your mind take center stage. For a couple of moments, be within the vastness and silence of your mind, viewing it from all angles, as if you were in the desert, looking up at the nighttime sky full of stars. Witness the sea of stars all around you. Every star is like a nerve cell in your mind, populating it with their radiance and brilliance. Scan your mind slowly, from left to right, looking for any places that are particularly dim or less illuminated with starlight, and if you find any dark spaces, with the power of your intention, fill them with new, fresh stars. Apply the stars liberally, without abandon. Make sure that there is an evenness to the sprinkle of stars in the sky of your mind.

Sitting back and reflecting, you take a deep breath in, and as you do, direct your breath to the millions of stars above you. Notice how they become brighter and even more radiant. With each subsequent breath, the stars become even more brilliant. Now there is almost more starshine than dark space in your mind.

And as the stars become infused with light with each passing breath, you begin to notice streams of light radiating from them and connecting them with each other. Each beam of light seems to intersect with other beams in the sky, and, soon, overhead, you see a network, a net of stars, that goes beyond mere constellations. You see that every star is truly linked to the others, like all the neurons in your mind are connected through their outstretched limbs and transferring information in a seamless manner. In the galaxy of your mind, there is cohesion, an interconnectedness that encompasses the space. You notice your thoughts flowing smoothly, gracefully, one star's light traveling to another, and the transfer of energy moves freely and with increasing momentum. The collective halo of the starlight forms the brilliance of your brain, the workings of your mind. Your mental functions—learning, decision-making, and remembering—become shiny and crystalline, glowing strong.

With a soft smile on your face, allow the curtains of your eyelids to rise up slowly, and you come back into the present moment of your daily life. If there is anything you want to remember for the future, make sure you associate that fact, face, or situation with a specific star in your mind so you can find it at any time you decide to go within.

Meditation: Every time there is something you want to remember, imagine your mind as a library of little wooden boxes. Allow the fact to come to your mind's eye to be imprinted, and then let it travel to one of the little wooden boxes. Remember the box's precise location so you can retrieve it at any time.

Menopause

Physical description: The cessation of menstruation (and, hence, fertility), defined as a lack of menstrual periods for twelve consecutive months. Typically occurs naturally at around age fifty. Menopausal symptoms include hot flashes, sleep disturbance, mood swings, vaginal dryness, thinning hair and skin, and increased fat deposition.

Energy center(s): Sacral, third eye

Nourishment: *Diet*—(1) Eat a diet abundant in plant foods, particularly those high in phytoestrogens, or weak plant estrogens, including soybeans, flaxseed meal and oil, nuts, whole grains, legumes, parsley, and fennel. (Please note that phytoestrogens are considered mildly estrogenic and may not be suitable for individuals with hormone-sensitive cancers. Check with your healthcare professional as to whether phytoestrogen-containing foods would be appropriate for you.); (2) Avoid or limit caffeine, spicy foods, alcohol, animal-based foods (meat), and refined carbohydrates. *Supplements*—(1) Vitamin C and bioflavonoids (e.g., quercetin, hesperidin) for capillary integrity; (2) Hormone-balancing botanicals, such as black cohosh, licorice, dong quai, and chasteberry.

Emotion(s): Fear, insecurity, anxiety

Limiting belief(s): I serve no purpose. My life force is dried up. My essence is connected to my ability to produce. What good am I?

Power animal: Snake

Flower essence(s): Chestnut Bud, Hornbeam, Mariposa Lily, Morning Glory

Affirmation(s): I live in the spirit of transformation. I create alchemy and healing in all that I do. I am reborn. I embody the mystical wisdom from my experiences.

Visualization: The moment you close your eyes you are connected to ribbons of a melody. The sound is sweet and has your essence, the sound of your soul, embedded within it. You are swept away by its light, mystical nature, and you follow it with your mind's eye. It arises

like tendrils of wispy smoke from the core of your heart and surrounds you, enveloping you in its everlasting purity. It brings you to
far off places—places on this planet you may have visited and that you
had a special, heartfelt connection to. The melody also takes you into
the layers of existence, into the fabric of the tapestry of all wisdom.
You follow the melody until you see a star- and gem-studded doorway before you. Seven stairs lead up to the doorway, which is filled
with a blinding white light.

Before you move farther, you stand back to take in this marvelous sight. The array of stars built into the doorway is bright, and their
beams of light funnel down to make a walkway to the entrance. The
gems—rubies, emeralds, sapphires, and diamonds—make an intricate pattern that weaves in and out of the star-studded structure.
They sparkle their essence forth in all directions: Rubies radiate the
strength of red, the essence of life and blood. Emeralds emit their
healing green light of nurturing. Sapphires spill forth their streams of
wisdom, and diamonds cast their beams of understanding and hope.
You stand there, soaking in all the vibrations of the gems, letting them
infuse your body, energy meridians, and chakras. Then you climb the
steps one by one—number one, number two, number three, num-
ber four, number five, number six, and finally, number seven, where
you pause to bask in the divine white light that pours forth from the
doorway.

As you step into the light, walking through the doorway, you realize that you are making an incredible transition into another realm.
Your body and soul are flooded with the energy of transformation
and alchemy. Your creativity has been morphed from the body, and
its essence, harbored in the ovaries and uterus, now weaves its way
through every cell of your being in the form of tiny, cool droplets of
dew. You see your body evolving into one that is intricately energized
and swirling with the creative potential of liberation. Tiny energetic
tendrils of your creative spirit spread out like lace throughout your
whole body, concentrating in the areas of your chakras and generating outward—rivulets of energy moving amongst your cells. This
transformative process takes place with menopause, the change of
life, moving you from a period of the expression of childbirth to a
period of the expression of your ultimate, overall creative potential.

On this side of the doorway, there are blossoming cherry trees
and an endless array of flowers—tulips, orchids, irises, lilies, sunflow-

ers, daisies, roses of all colors, magnolias, pansies, gladiolas, and poppies. They line your path, extending out as far as the eye can see. You welcome this change of life, feeling free, connecting to your creativity, and blossoming to your inner alchemy.

Meditation: Journal on how you would like to redefine yourself in this next phase of your life. What do you want to cultivate? How do you align all parts of yourself in harmony?

Menstrual Difficulties

Physical description: Mild or severe symptoms felt before, during, or after a woman's menstrual period, including abdominal pain or cramps, lower backache, bloating, breast tenderness, mood changes, nausea, fatigue, heavy bleeding, and the presence of excessive blood clots.

Energy center(s): Sacral, third eye

Nourishment: *Diet*—(1) Eat a diet consisting of primarily unprocessed, whole plant foods (and containing low or negligible amounts of animal-based foods, like meat); (2) Avoid or limit caffeine, alcohol, and refined carbohydrates. *Supplements*—(1) Omega-3 fatty-acid (from flax or fish oil) supplement to balance inflammatory prostaglandin production; (2) Iron supplement if iron-deficiency exists due to heavy bleeding; (3) Calcium-magnesium supplement for cramps, muscle aches, and anxiety; (4) B-complex vitamin for stress reduction.

Emotion(s): Vulnerability, jealousy, competition

Limiting belief(s): I reject my femininity. I resist the male figures in my life. I refuse my sexuality. My inner nature is imbalanced. My life feels stagnant, like a dead end. I attract difficulties. I feel out of touch with my intuition. I strive to survive.

Power animal: Beaver

Flower essence(s): Alpine Lily, Chamomile, Easter Lily, Holly, Morning Glory, St. John's Wort

Affirmation(s): The feminine and masculine within me dance with harmony. I am fertile with possibilities and creativity. I flow with ease. I am open to my psychic self.

Visualization: Cup your hands in a bowl-like formation and rest them at the base of your belly, in the creases between your legs and torso. Create a healing receptacle through your hands. In your mind's eye, see a durable copper bowl resting within your low abdomen. This bowl is big enough that it spans the length of your pelvis, and it is as deep as the distance from your navel to the bottom of your pelvic basin. Perceive this bowl as a sacred Tibetan bowl etched around the rim with ancient symbols and language that impart healing messages to your body. See those symbols dance from the bowl and into the matrix of your cells. Deep and full of wisdom, they become parts of you.

Your reproductive organs fit perfectly within this bowl structure. It is wide and deep enough to harbor your uterus, vagina, fallopian tubes, and ovaries. In some ways, the bowl almost feels like a protective shell, not only for your precious organs, but also for your femininity, creativity, and emotions. All is contained within the boundaries of this bowl. Any emotions that have been stored for an excessive period of time and need to come out feel safe enough to venture out of the structures of your body and into the holding space of the bowl.

Your sense of femininity, which has long been cloistered and packed away neatly, can arise gently from her slumber. She rises from the bowl like wisps of sacred smoke. The tendrils of smoke waft their way up into your nostrils, and you smell a sweet, sandalwood-and-rose aroma. The essence of your vulnerability, strength, and grace is embodied by the intertwining dance of these two scents.

And finally, your creativity dances to an internal beat that only you recognize. It begins its dance along the concave walls of the bowl, building momentum and vitality and vigor. There is a certain feeling of freshness, like dew on daffodils in spring, which washes over your internal self. At once, you feel renewed and vitalized by this movement within you. Your reproductive organs begin to vibrate with the motion of your creativity. Their dormant and even stagnant existence shakes loose with the freedom you feel from the liberation of your pure creativity. You have missed your connection to your creative self, and now you have it back again, flowing and strong. She pulses within you, steady, like the blood flowing through your veins.

At this moment, you are handed a wooden stick about six inches long and about one inch wide. You are instructed to move the stick in a clockwise fashion around the outer rim of the Tibetan bowl. Starting at the side closest to your spine, you position the stick upright and slowly begin swirling it around the rim of the bowl in the direction of the sun, and as you move it round and round, cyclically, you become mesmerized by the movement.

You increase the pace slightly, to the extent that the bowl begins to make a soft hum, but a hum that has incredible substance and depth. As you accelerate your stick's movement around the bowl, the resonance of the bowl becomes stronger, more pronounced, and the vibration of the sound begins to radiate from your low belly like the light of a star. Beams of vibration stream through your legs, your torso, your arms, and your head. These beams of starlight are, in turn, made of tiny stars, and the tiny stars are made of even smaller stars. In this perfect moment, you remember your perfect connection and unification with the universe.

The song of your Tibetan bowl releases and breaks up any stagnant patterns in your reproductive organs, sending them out to the universal void. The purity of the sound creates transformational movement within you, and all menstrual difficulties, including cramping, clotting, heavy bleeding, or abnormal periods, fall away from you like old skin shed from a snake. A vital energy takes its residence within your low belly and fills your uterus with pink light, which then flows to your fallopian tubes and ovaries. Your creativity is glowing, your femininity is thriving, and your emotions are unleashed and free.

Meditation: Meditate on the alignment of your sacral chakra with that of your third-eye chakra. See your low belly spinning outward and your third eye spiraling forward. Let both converge on a central point. Feel your feminine instinct and intuition blend together.

Migraines

Physical description: A severe, pulsating headache accompanied by nausea, vomiting, and sensitivity to light and sound.

Energy center(s): Third eye

Nourishment: *Diet*—(1) Work with a qualified healthcare professional to identify food allergies; (2) Avoid histamine-containing foods such as: chocolate, alcohol, cheese, citrus fruits, and shellfish; (3) Avoid or limit animal foods, as they are higher in inflammatory fats compared with plant foods; (4) Emphasize anti-inflammatory foods, such as ginger, turmeric (curries), onions, garlic, and fats from flaxseed oil and cold-water fish; (5) Eliminate processed foods containing food additives, refined sugar, caffeine, and excessive sodium. *Supplements*—(1) Magnesium for healthy nerve stimulation; (2) B-complex vitamin for reducing the impact of stress on body function; (3) Vitamin C and bioflavonoids for supporting the immune system, adrenals, and vasculature; (4) Botanical anti-inflammatories for migraines: feverfew, butterbur, ginger, and peppermint.

Emotion(s): Built-up tension, anger, or irritation

Limiting belief(s): I am going to blow my top! Anger pulses through me. I am overly sensitive to my environment.

Power animal: Polar bear

Flower essence(s): Aspen, Cherry Plum, Lavender

Affirmation(s): I am the loving observer of events around me. All mental tension melts like butter on a griddle. I am open to the messages of my insightful, sensitive nature.

Visualization: If you are having a migraine at this time, put your energy fully and completely into the throbbing, painful sensations in your skull. Let your whole self dive into the pain you feel. And while you are deep within the pain, observe the surroundings. What images do you see? What messages do you hear? What special significance do the images and messages carry for you in this migraine moment?

Now, staying with the pain and the surrounding images and sounds, take a luxurious, deep breath, breathing in a wave of comfort and light. As this healing breath travels into your nostrils, let it waft up through both nostrils simultaneously. The breath coming in the left nostril slowly moves up and over to the left temple, and the breath coming in the right nostril penetrates the space along the way to the right temple. These currents of comforting breath spiral in the temples, eventually going inward to meet in the center of your forehead.

Once the two streams of air meet in the middle, they form a small cloud of cool, healing condensation made of aquamarine-colored droplets. Each of these droplets is its own tiny spiral, and with your next breath, each one disperses through your entire head, like a mist, cooling down any inflammation and signaling to your immune system that it should relax and reduce any overactive responses. You can add to the droplets by sending your breath up your nostrils and feeding it into your temples, streaming the two sides together, creating more condensation, and adding to the cycle of droplet dispersal. You continue a couple more rounds of this activity, moving the droplets through your mind, easing any pain or throbbing, and eventually you feel a release of these sensations.

Place your hands on either side of your head and envision them as being magnets. Let all the excess cooling droplets magnetize to your hands. Wait until your hands feel heavy and then put them together, moving them gently back and forth to create warmth and the healing energy of the fire element in your hands.

From there, take both hands to the front of your scalp and slowly move them through your hair to the back of your head, letting all the energy from your hands seal in the healing within your head. At once, you feel an opening and expansiveness in your head rather than a tightness and constriction. Peeking into your head through your mind's eye, you set your gaze upon a vision of blue sky—open, without obstruction. The brilliance of the crown chakra filters through the top of your head like radiant sunshine permeating the expanse of sky. And with a grateful heart, you give thanks for the release of your migraine pain.

Meditation: Sit in silence with your fingers in the fire-earth mudra (a specific finger position) to balance these elements within you. For each hand, touch your thumb to your middle finger. Imagine the harmonious circulation of these energies through your body.

Morning Sickness (See Nausea)

Motion Sickness (See Nausea)

Multiple Sclerosis

Physical description: An autoimmune condition in which the body's inherent immune system attacks the central nervous system, specifically the sheath coatings around nerves, referred to as myelin. With disrupted myelin, the body can no longer effectively transmit signals through the nervous system. Physical disability and mental functioning decline as a result.

Energy center(s): Root, crown

Nourishment: *Diet*—(1) Reduce or eliminate animal foods (except for cold-water fish) as much as possible; (2) Work with a qualified healthcare professional to identify food allergies; (3) Emphasize organically grown produce whenever possible. *Supplements*—(1) A high-quality, high-potency multivitamin and mineral; (2) Omega-3 fats (from fish or flaxseed oil); (3) Digestive enzymes in between meals; (4) Assess blood levels of vitamin D and supplement if deficient.

Emotion(s): Fear of exposure, vulnerability, nervousness, insecurity, inadequacy

Limiting belief(s): I feel unsupported and vulnerable. I am unable to transform impulse into action. My body and spirit are fragmented and imbalanced.

Power animal: Ram

Flower essence(s): Angelica, Chamomile, Crab Apple, Forget-me-not, Mallow

Affirmation(s): I transmit love and radiance through every part of my body. The essence of my being is unified and in alignment with all of life. I welcome new beginnings.

Visualization: With your eyes closed and your body at rest, imagine a large spiral of gold and silver before your mind's eye. Every breath you take follows the same rhythm as the movement of the spiral—nice and slow, but also solid and assured. Seeing this shining spiral before you relaxes you completely.

Take a deep breath in, allowing the abundant source of oxygen to travel to your tailbone. When you are ready, exhale fully while at the same time imagining the breath leaving your body through the top of your head. With each subsequent breath, see the column of breath travel from your tail to your head, clearing any residue or blocks. You begin to feel light and invigorated; any heaviness or worn feeling is released, to be carried out on the vehicle of the breath.

Now invite the large, circulating spiral to slip over you like a sheath. You stand in the middle of the spiral, captivated with love by its protective radiance. You feel as though you have been blanketed in a secure feeling of safety. Every part of you is protected, cushioned, softened. No situation in your life feels the least bit threatening. You sink into this safety further, letting your body relax even more. Your shoulders pull away from your ears; your chest expands wider to allow more breath to travel into your lungs. Your belly softens to receive the breath, and your legs and feet tingle with the flow of more blood and oxygen.

The spiral continues its motion around your being, and you stay connected to its rhythm with your cleansing and nourishing breath. The winding gold and silver strands of the spiral, capturing the essence of yang and yin, action and inaction, infuse your being to create balance in all your organ systems, particularly in your immune and nervous systems. Your entire body feels harmonious, loving, and peaceful.

As you take a generous, long breath, the spiral around you becomes smaller, about the length of your spinal column, and begins to weave itself around your spine, starting at your tailbone and continuing slowly and lovingly around your spine. It rises up the middle spine to the upper spine and coats your brain with the essence of the protective yang and yin, permeating all of your nerve cells. Your entire central nervous system feels full of integrity and strength. Any damage to your nervous system has been repaired through the healing action of the spiral, which now coats your spinal column and all of your precious nerves residing in your brain tissue. Your body is glowing with the bliss of being balanced and complete.

Meditation: In your meditation, visualize a protective coating over your entire being. Invite this spiritual sheath to envelop you as you infuse the secured area with the radiance of the color gold. Bask in the glow of your illuminated self.

Muscle Tightness

Physical description: A tense, stiff, uncomfortable feeling in certain muscles due to physical and/or psychological stress(ors).

Energy center(s): Root

Nourishment: *Diet*—(1) Drink adequate fluids; (2) Eat an alkalizing diet high in nonstarchy vegetables, particularly green, leafy vegetables and sprouts. *Supplements*—(1) A high-quality multivitamin and mineral; (2) Additional magnesium, calcium, and potassium.

Emotion(s): Tension, worry, fear

Limiting belief(s): I am exposed. I am unsupported. I harbor all tension.

Power animal: Elk

Flower essence(s): Cherry Plum, Dogwood, Echinacea, Elm, Star of Bethlehem, Willow

Affirmation(s): I am held in the loving grace of the universe. I release to the earth all that serves me incorrectly. My muscles are loose, limber, and nourished with every movement. I endure any difficulty with the strength that resides in my fibers.

Visualization: Close your eyes. Let go into the moment as much as you possibly can. Imagine you are flying like a bird, high in an aquamarine sky. You are light and flowing, having shed all worry, pain, and preoccupation. Breathe in with awareness and trust, and exhale your breath through to your outstretched arms, releasing to the infinite universe. Use your breath to carry you in flight: the inhale serves as a means to make you more buoyant, and the exhale is a way to make you glide effortlessly throughout the clear, beautiful space surrounding you. You remember feeling a peace like this long ago. And now your present everyday life feels cluttered, busy, and tense. As you surrender to the expanse of sky, you wonder how you could have arrived at the place of tension that you have found yourself in.

You fly to a comfortable resting place so you can lie down and go deeper into the landscape of your body to find any residual places of tension. Allowing your body to relax as best you can, you decide to scan your muscles to see whether they are holding any worry, tightness, or stress that needs to be dissolved so you can move more gracefully throughout your days. You start at the top of your body, at your head, and you bring in the cleansing, clearing element of air, allowing this gentle breeze to circulate through all of your face and head, expanding and releasing any tightness.

You may observe that you hold your tension around your eyes, in your cheeks, in your temples, around your jaw, and even in your neck muscles. With the smooth circulation of air that fills the pure sky, you fill every muscle fiber with small spirals of current. Immediately, you feel a release in any places that felt tight.

You guide this air spiral down to your chest and back. You see that you carry many places of tension within your torso. Put your awareness into these places, guiding the streaming current of warm air through every ribbon of muscle fiber, warming and expanding it.

With each tension release, you feel more and more energy coming into your body.

Ripple this warm air into places in your back—your upper back, mid back, and low back—and feel your back sink into the ground beneath it, trusting that it is protected. Your back feels more loose and limber than it has in a long time.

Follow this relaxing current into your legs. Allow both legs to fill with several lines of streaming warm air, which penetrates the deep, layered muscle fibers, and let your legs go soft, like jelly. Any and all tightness melts and flies away into the current of air. No tension remains behind, and your legs feel light and feathery as the wisp of air exits out your feet.

You become aware of just how much tension your body was holding, and you vow to yourself to remember to always come back to this feeling of lightness and airiness, reminding yourself of your freedom. See all of your muscles becoming nourished by the energy of your subsequent breaths. Any time you feel any tension, use your breath to circulate the current of the sky through the tension and liberate it. And now you are free to fly once again.

Open your eyes slowly while, at the same time, filling yourself with compassion for your physical body. Rotate your neck slowly. Wiggle your arms gently. Move your torso from side to side. Shift your legs back and forth, and rock your feet to and fro. Give thanks to your muscles for their capacity to act as shock absorbers, and give them permission to let go of any shocks that hold them back.

Meditation: Treat yourself to a soothing, reflective, meditative bath with Epsom salts (one to two cups) and baking soda (one cup).

Myopia (See Nearsightedness)

Nausea (Morning Sickness, Motion Sickness)

Physical description: A feeling of uneasiness that is associated with the urge to vomit.

Energy center(s): Solar plexus, throat

Nourishment: *Diet*—(1) Keep blood sugar stable by eating small, frequent snacks/meals throughout the day, particularly before bedtime and after waking; (2) Ginger tea. *Supplements*—Ginger-root extract.

Emotion(s): Uneasiness, refusal, denial

Limiting belief(s): I am uneasy about the situation. I refuse to accept and assimilate _____ (fill in the blank—an event, a person's actions, the presence of a person).

Power animal: Dragonfly

Flower essence(s): Honeysuckle, Rabbitbrush, Walnut, Willow

Affirmation(s): I am filled with loving comfort. All events are integrated within my being in a way that is beneficial for who I am. I accept to the extent I can in this moment.

Visualization: Steady yourself with the anchor of your breath. Breathe in deeply and pull the fresh oxygen down to your belly. With each inhale, guide yourself to stillness; each breath lights the path in that direction. As you collect deep breaths in the pit of your belly, see them gradually accumulate to create a quiet, peaceful place about the size of your hand and that you can sink into. It is enclosed like a bubble. With every ounce of your awareness, move into this enclosed, safe space that is devoid of any outside distractions or discomfort. It is the single place in your being that you feel completely grounded and centered and free of nausea. Call it the "still point."

Make this still-point bubble larger using the vehicle of your breath. With each inhale, you add more room to the already formed bubble. And with the next breath, you add still more room. Continue adding room until you have rippled stillness throughout all your limbs, your torso, and your head. The vibration of the ripples of stillness cast out any feeling of uneasiness or upset.

Take your time to engage with the still-point bubble thoroughly and completely. By the time you have finished connecting to and creating it through your breath, you will notice that your entire being is relaxed, centered, and free of any nausea.

Meditation: Meditate on your still point.

Nearsightedness (Myopia)

Physical description: An inability to see objects at a distance

Energy center(s): Third eye

Nourishment: *Diet*—(1) Eat foods high in the yellow plant pigment lutein, such as green, leafy vegetables (spinach is a good source); (2) Include dietary sources of omega-3 fats, such as fish, leafy greens, nuts, and seeds (e.g., flaxseed meal or oil). *Supplements*—A high-quality multivitamin and mineral containing vitamins A, C, and E and zinc.

Emotion(s): Fear of what lays ahead, of the unknown

Limiting belief(s): I fear moving forward into the unknown. I refuse to focus my attention on goals because I fear failure. I am set in my comfortable ways.

Power animal: Eagle

Flower essence(s): Filaree, Queen Anne's Lace, Shasta Daisy

Affirmation(s): I embrace healthy risks and challenges. I successfully integrate the big picture of life and the details of my everyday living. My inner and outer visions are aligned. I see clearly.

Visualization: Close your eyes. Rub your hands together briskly until they become a little bit warm from the friction, and cup both of your eyes simultaneously, letting the energy from your hands invigorate your eyes. Imagine the energy moves into each eye through the lens and into the body of the eye, all the way to the back of the eye (called the retina). See the spectrum of energy moving inward very point-edly—almost as if in each cupped palm you held a small diamond prism reflecting a beam of rainbow light—and precisely through your eye.

Now imagine the beam of light moves upward. Follow its path with your eyes. Stretch your eye muscles by focusing upward and outward as far as feels comfortable. And now see the beam of light move down, stretching your eyes in the opposite direction to follow it. Bring your eyes back to a neutral position and see the beam of rainbow light before you. Move your eyes to the left this time, following the trail of light from the prism. And then move in the opposite direction—to the right—as the beam of light shifts its path. Bring your eyes back to neutral, in the center, and focus on the prisms in both hands. Repeat this eye-stretching exercise if you like, if you think that your eyes need more relaxation.

Once your gaze is fixed forward into the prisms, let them become your magnifiers for objects in the distance. Let the prism impart to your eyes the qualities of sharpness, focus, detail, and directness. It removes all obstructions to you seeing faraway objects and clears away all fears about the past, present, and future. All images that are directed into your eyes move past the lens in the front and fall perfectly on to the back of your eye so objects can be seen at a distance with amazing clarity. Remove your hands from your eyes and place this affirmation, in written text, somewhere in your visual field on a daily basis: "I see clearly."

Meditation: Allow your eyes to relax, and gently fix your gaze on an object in the distance. As you focus on this object, contemplate what you fear in your near and distant future. Why do you fear it? How can you see it more clearly for what it is?

Neck Pain

Physical description: Sharp or dull pain or stiffness in the neck that can limit function.

Energy center(s): Throat

Nourishment: *Diet*—(1) Drink adequate fluids; (2) Eat an alkalizing diet high in nonstarchy vegetables, particularly green, leafy vegetables and sprouts. *Supplements*—(1) A high-quality multivitamin and mineral; (2) Additional magnesium, calcium, and potassium in a supplement.

Emotion(s): Fear, feeling stifled

Limiting belief(s): Life is a pain in the neck. My true self suffers. I am burdened. Something is holding me back.

Power animal: Swan

Flower essence(s): Elm, Fairy Lantern, Lady's Slipper

Affirmation(s): My heart releases my passions through the canal of my neck. I choose to live life in an authentic way. I release myself from burdens and pains, and I welcome healing and choice in their place. I am supported. I hold my head high and face the world.

Visualization: Gently cradle your neck in your hands while you feel your breath repeatedly sinking into you and escaping from you. Feel the heaviness and pain in your neck. Let them speak to you. Listen to them carefully, as their voices have not been heard. What do they say? Thank them for giving you this information, for giving you a sign that you may have felt a lack of support, an inability to choose and to put together, which makes life feel like drudgery. Allow their concerns to be heard and then evaporate. With each concern that they share, the voices of the heaviness and pain become quieter until finally they dissolve, melting away like butter and leaving your neck supple and soft, free of any obstruction or pain.

Take a breath in, and visualize it as the color of a bright blue sky. As you inhale this sky energy, extend its essence and vastness throughout the terrain of your neck. It helps you to open and expand your neck, allowing you to tilt your head to the sky. And when you peer into the sky, you are reminded of the infinity of choices in your life. Every cloud that sails by returns you to the easygoing nature of living. The tightness and armor around your neck has fallen off, and now you are free and light. You watch the sky turn from light blue to a deep indigo, revealing a universe filled with stars that sit in the heavens like diamonds. They sparkle, serving as another reminder of the many facets of your life, and how they shine depends on how you see them.

Now take a deep sigh, tilting your head slightly downward, so that your inner gaze is focused in the middle of your chest, at the heart. Your beautiful heart is bundled up in many layers, like an onion. It calls you to unravel it, to explore its depths. Gently, you begin peeling back the intricate layers of your heart, and as you do so, a cacophony of whispers is released. Your passions are unveiled. All of your dreams, your sense of purpose, your talents, and gifts—hiding within the layers of the heart, buried deep, remaining unexpressed—are now revealed. You choose to honor them by letting them float upwards to the neck, releasing them to the world in the form of your resonant voice and meaningful words. Allow yourself to say whatever needs to come forward. Then give thanks to your neck for being the vehicle for your authentic self. Finally, you promise to yourself to continue the exploration and discovery of your heart field, and its fruits of passions, dreams, and expressions, throughout your daily living, giving your neck the support it needs to allow their release.

Meditation: Meditate on the color of a bright blue sky, releasing your tension to the clouds floating freely overhead.

Numbness

Physical description: A lack of sensation

Energy center(s): Crown

Nourishment: *Diet*—(1) Balance blood sugar by eating foods that have a low glycemic index, such as legumes, whole grains, nonstarchy vegetables, and lean meats; (2) Drink adequate fluids; (3) Avoid foods high in fat, refined carbohydrates, food additives, and caffeine; (4) Eat organically grown foods as much as possible. *Supplements*—(1) Acetyl-L-carnitine; (2) Alpha-lipoic acid; (3) Unsaturated fats: gamma linolenic acid, eicosapentaenoic acid, docosahexaenoic acid; (4) B-complex vitamin (especially biotin, vitamin B6).

Emotion(s): Distance, coldness, rejection, fear

Limiting belief(s): I close myself off because of fear. It is safer for me to be distant from others. I am untrusting of my body's messages.

Power animal: Leopard

Flower essence(s): California Pitcher Plant, Indian Pink, Mugwort, Oregon Grape, Star Tulip

Affirmation(s): I move into the mystery with my full self. My feelings provide me with the insight and instinct to act. I cherish my body's messages.

Visualization: Close your eyes. Relax as much as you are able to in the moment. In your mind's eye, see yourself standing before you as a being in armor, similar to that of a medieval knight. You have a thick shell to your being, particularly in the areas of your body where you feel numbness.

Ask the numb parts of yourself what they are trying to say. What do you have a lack of feeling about, or where do you need more feeling in your life? With your perked, attentive, intuitive ears, listen carefully to what they say to you. As they speak their wisdom, the heavily armored layers start to peel off you, falling to the ground beside you and shattering. They shatter into small pieces of metal that sift into the soil to become nourishment for the earth.

Begin to see what lies underneath the armor. Put your attention on the many alive, colorful, active layers that compose your true self. These multicolored layers are delicate and responsive to the flow of actions, thoughts, emotions, and beliefs running through your body like pieces of thin soft silk rippling in the breeze. See your higher consciousness streaming through the energy meridian superhighway that is interlaced throughout your body. It pushes any obstacles out of the way and opens doorways of solutions to challenges. In this moment, you have become a fluid, harmonized being full of sensation. You can feel yourself becoming invigorated and active with the pulsation of life.

The pulse of life now ripples through each of your energy meridians, entering through your head, coursing through the body, and exiting through either the hands or feet. The flow of your higher consciousness and the pulse of life swirl together in your extremities, purging all remaining residual blocks and stagnation through each fingertip of both hands—thumb, forefinger, middle finger, ring finger, and baby finger. See your fingers become electric with the pulse of life and very sensitive to their surroundings. Imagine the same happening through the feet; more blocks and stagnation release from both feet simultaneously, starting in the big toes and moving through the second toes, third toes, fourth, and fifth. Your energy is running clearly and smoothly throughout your body.

Meditation: Examine your five senses—touch, taste, hearing, sight, smell—by dedicating an entire week to creating awareness about that particular sense. Perhaps you start the first week with smell. Become sensitive to all smells, odors, aromas, and fragrances around you. What feelings do they provoke? Continue with the remaining senses and see which one you've been most relying upon and which one you've been depending on least.

Obesity (See Overweight)

Osteoarthritis

Physical description: A progressive, degenerative disease of the joints in which there is a loss of cartilage, resulting in joint stiffness, pain, and impaired function.

Energy center(s): Root

Nourishment: *Diet*—(1) Emphasize anti-inflammatory, plant-based foods (fruits, vegetables, cold-water fish, legumes, whole grains) in place of an inflammatory, meat-based diet; (2) Test whether a nightshade-free diet is beneficial for symptom relief by eliminating tomatoes, potatoes, peppers (all kinds), and eggplant. *Supplements*—(1) A high-quality, high-potency multivitamin and mineral; (2) Digestive enzymes (e.g., bromelain) in between meals; (3) Joint-supporting nutrients such as glucosamine and chondroitin; (4) Anti-inflammatory botanicals like boswellia, ginger, curcumin, and bioflavonoids (e.g., quercetin).

Emotion(s): Resentment, anger, bitterness, stagnation, criticalness

Limiting belief(s): I feel, stuck, stagnant, and out of control. Anger and bitterness immobilize me. My need for control and structure makes me rigid and immobile.

Power animal: Antelope

Flower essence(s): Dogwood, Larch, Pine

Affirmation(s): I am free and flowing with the river of life. I let go of any event or emotion that serves me incorrectly. I release any past pain or irritation. I adapt easily.

Visualization: Close your eyes and in your mind's eye, see your entire body in its current state before you. Use your built-in, special, intuitive vision that detects emotional scars, wounds, and trauma to scan this body image, starting with the head, from top to bottom. Look within your entire skull for any stagnant, stuck thoughts that have been lodged inside your brain, repeating themselves over and over, making you unable to move forward in a healthy way. See these thoughts fly from your head the moment you uncover them. These thoughts instantly become transformed into birds, flying high in the sky, basking in their freedom. Your mind feels clearer, and you are engulfed in a sense of release from the burden of these negative thoughts. Breathe deeply and let yourself be washed over with a renewed sense of peace.

Now use your inner vision to scan your neck, shoulders, arms, and fingers. See if there are any blocks, burdens, or energy you have been carrying or taking in that makes you feel heavy and stiff. If there are, allow them to melt away like butter, dripping down from your neck, cascading down your shoulders, rolling down your arms, and exiting through your fingertips. These parts of you are instantaneously infused with a feeling of golden lightness. Every bone in this part of your body is radiating with the essence of a carefree life. You can see the body image before you happily shake out its shoulders, arms, and hands. Each finger appears to have been dipped in the gold of the flowing sunshine that floods your being. The fingers no longer clutch to the past or try to control the future.

From here, you travel into your torso, scanning your way down from your heart into your lungs and, from there, finally, into the many tubes of your digestive tract. Along the way, note very carefully whether there are any stuck, tarlike places within your torso, and shine a laser of pure white light to break them up into little fragments. These fragments transform from their black sludge into tiny crystals that shine and sparkle throughout your body. Once you are done with applying the laser to the image of your torso, your heart is sparkling like a large diamond; your lungs are like opalescent containers, receiving your energetic breath; and your digestive system is smooth and glossy with a flowing, luminescent liquid that purifies all that you take in. This liquid sloshes and swirls in the pelvic basin and permeates the hipbone, making it supple and flexible once again. It descends into the bones of the legs, invigorating your thighs, knees, and calves. Your lower body is alight with the ability to move freely, without irritation, pain, swelling, or stiffness.

The image of you before your mind's eye is streaming with white light that has removed all obstacles to your wellness. Step into this healed image and become this transformed version of yourself, which is free from osteoarthritis. Open your eyes to your new self!

Meditation: Meditate on the words *support, nourishment,* and *movement.* At the end of the meditation, string them together into an affirmation that resonates with you.

Osteoporosis

Physical description: A bone disorder in which the bone thins and loses density and, as a result, becomes more prone to fracture.

Energy center(s): Root

Nourishment: *Diet*—(1) Eat a diet abundant in alkalizing, non-starchy vegetables, especially green, leafy vegetables and fruits; (2) Avoid or limit acidifying animal-based products, such as meats and cheeses, as well as other foods like salt, sugar, soft drinks, alcohol, and coffee. *Supplements*—(1) Calcium taken together with vitamin D (to enhance absorption of calcium in the gut). Take calcium in small doses throughout the day, with the largest dose before bedtime; (2) A general multimineral supplement; (3) Vitamin K.

Emotion(s): Feeling fragile, resentment, vulnerability

Limiting belief(s): My beliefs have been chiseled away; the root of my being is brittle, and my trust is thin. I have had experiences that have poked holes in the foundation of my being. My ability to trust and connect to the physical world feels fragile.

Power animal: Antelope

Flower essence(s): Baby Blue Eyes, Dogwood, Gorse, Oregon Grape, Scleranthus

Affirmation(s): I am solid, steady, and strong in my foundation, yet flexible and yielding—all in the proper proportion for my highest self. The strength within me moves me forward with confidence.

Visualization: In your own time, when you feel ready and safe, close your eyes and take a relaxing breath. Note the positioning of your feet; make sure they are planted firmly on the ground and that your legs are uncrossed if you are sitting down. Position your arms at either side of your body, allowing them to be free and dangle or to rest upon your thighs if you are sitting.

With your mind's eye, magnify your inner gaze downwards into the earth's crust. Imagine you have a special vision capability to see through the crust. Observe the dense, abundant mineral content of the earth layer by layer. See how ribbons of minerals are embedded in and laced through its structure, all in a perfect, harmonious blend for the earth. Envision these minerals as providing the skeleton for the planet.

While you let yourself go into that image, tap into the strength and solidity of the earth beneath you. Connect with the skeleton of the earth and unify your energy with her energy, seeing the earth as a living, breathing organism—Gaia. Let appreciation come forth from your heart for her ability to encompass and share the elements of air, metal, water, and fire. Feel those elements within her through the connection you have with her in your feet. Invite the elements to circle and circulate in the souls of your feet, in a pinwheel-like fashion, moving slowly and thoroughly. In particular, draw the symbolic element of metal, which harbors all the important soft metals in a perfect ratio for your bones, up into your skeleton. Thread the solid, yet flexible energy of these earth minerals into the matrix of your bones. See your bones filling up like a glass filling with opaque, thick milk. Let the mineral mixture deposit itself onto the latticelike matrix of your bone tissue, like concrete being poured into the iron-wrought foundation for a house. Allow all of the minerals to seep into your bone, coating it and filling any cracks, holes, or small pores in with the dense energy of the minerals. Let your bones feel this difference. Put your awareness completely in your skeleton. How do your bones feel? What sensations do you notice?

Using the creativity of your mind's eye, envision your skeleton from a point outside of your body, so you are viewing your skeleton in front of you. See it as free and flexible, able to move and glide and walk gracefully and confidently. Look closer into your bone tissue and see how dynamic it is, responding to movement and momentum, being stimulated through weight-bearing activities like walking or lifting weights. Envision your skeleton being active, and at the same time it is active, notice how your bone cells become invigorated. They work to support your movement by making more bone cells.

Using your inner microscope, magnify the bone tissue. See your bone-forming cells in perfect balance with your bone-breakdown cells. Their activity is healthy and makes your bones resistant to disease or fracture.

And even though your bones feel strong, notice how flexible they also are. The matrix of the bone allows it to be yielding and responsive to movement, while the minerals give your bones an excellent balance of density and firmness.

Take a breath, and as you do so, feel your body fully anchored into the template of your skeleton. Let your muscles hug your skeleton, and let all the joints be flexible and flowing.

And with a final breath, envision a beam of white light coming in through the soles of your feet, running like white columns up your legs, giving you the feeling that you are standing on two strong pillars. Guide the light up into your hipbones, your spinal column, your ribs, and arms, and lastly, shine this brilliant light into the skull. This light seals in all the healing that has been imparted to you from the earth.

Take a gentle breath in, wiggle your toes, and open your eyes.

Meditation: Invigorate and stimulate your bones with a weight-bearing meditative activity. Take a leisurely walk in the sun (so you can get some vitamin D), and as you do, contemplate each step you take. See each step as significant and strengthening. Make the movement your sole focus.

Ovarian Cysts (Polycystic Ovarian Syndrome)

Physical description: Fluid-filled sacs found in the ovaries which may cause bleeding, pain, or discomfort.

Energy center(s): Sacral

Nourishment: *Diet*—Balance blood sugar by eating small, frequent snacks/meals throughout the day in addition to eating high-fiber, low-glycemic-index foods such as legumes, whole grains, non starchy vegetables, and fruits. *Supplements*—(1) A high-quality multi-vitamin/mineral; (2) Inositol; (3) Blood sugar balancing supplements such as chromium, cinnamon, and green tea extract.

Emotion(s): Fear, doubt about ability

Limiting belief(s): My creativity proliferates inside me. I hold back on expressing my true, creative self. My ideas are not heard or implemented. My femininity remains dormant.

Power animal: Crow

Flower essence(s): Indian Paintbrush, Tansy, Tiger Lily

Affirmation(s): I accept and welcome my creative potential to the degree that it serves me in good, true, and beautiful ways. I am abundant with creative ideas that I express to others. The feminine part of my self blossoms abundantly and beautifully.

Visualization: Find stillness within you and see if you can locate it deep within your low abdomen, at the level of your ovaries, which sit on the low left and right sides, tucked in a bit from your pelvis. Breathe grace into this place of creation and beauty, and give your femininity permission to blossom outward, like a lily opening. Observe what lives in this space of you. Do you see images, colors, people? Or do you hear sounds?

Imagine energy being smoothed, like warm melted butter, over your low abdomen, allowing your abdomen to expand even more so you can examine the many layers inside.

With your heart, view your left ovary. Notice any messages that it has for you. The creative potential of your ovaries is tremendous and constantly being stimulated. Sometimes they ask you to explore ideas, new opinions, and novel creations. What "growths" do you have here? What is it encouraging you to uncover and discover? Are there aspects that need to come to light? Take some time to allow complete answers to these questions to come through.

Pause here for a couple of seconds or minutes.

The water element resonates to the energy of the ovaries. Envision a small, cascading waterfall of pink and gold light to fall upon the left ovary, bringing it back into balance and restoring its creative potential to a level that suits your body and spirit. Continue to let the pink and yellow light swirl through, in a circular motion, within your left ovary. If there is anything that needs releasing, let it fall into the waterfall of energy and be carried away. Enjoy a deep breath of confidence and reassurance here. Anchor the breath into the fertile ground of the left ovary.

Once you feel a clearing in the left ovary, walk your heart consciousness over to your right ovary. With an ear bent in this direction, listen with an attentive heart to what your right ovary has to say to you at this time.

Pause briefly.

After you have taken some time to listen, ask some of your own questions: What wants action in your life? What part of your life is craving motion or movement and a release from stagnation? Are your masculine and feminine energies in balance? Do you feel safe being fully feminine, organic, and creative, or do you feel stifled, oppressed, particularly by men in your life? Watch for what reveals itself. How do you feel about these answers or responses?

When you are satisfied with your experience here, invite the pink and gold waterfall of energy to begin flowing down into the right ovary, ungluing any stuckness or indecision, or any outdated patterns around what it means to be a woman. Open yourself to the spiraling, clearing pink and gold energy moving around your right ovary in a clockwise manner.

When you feel that the process has completed, rest your left hand on your left ovary and your right hand on your right ovary. Gently move your torso side to side, feeling the sway of movement back and forth, from left to right and right to left. Shift your movement into one that is circular and subtle, and as you move, see the pink and gold energy painting your insides of your low belly. In an instant, you are overcome with a relaxing sensation, fully alive and vibrant, and at the same time, accepting every aspect of who you are as a woman. The pink and gold energy washes away any overgrowths or imbalances in your ovaries, bringing you to a state of pure balance.

Bring your body to rest, your hands at the sides of your body, and affirm to yourself, "I accept and welcome my creative potential to the degree that it serves me in good, true, and beautiful ways."

Meditation: Ensure that your creativity is nourished and expressed by keeping a journal specifically for all the creative ideas you have.

Overweight (Obesity)

Physical description: The body has accumulated too much fat mass for its stature, to the point that an unhealthy physiology, such as limited function, inflammation, and metabolic disturbance, has been created.

Energy center(s): Root, sacral, solar plexus, heart, throat, third eye, crown

Nourishment: *Diet*—(1) Eat fewer calories; (2) Eat slowly and mindfully. Refrain from eating when you are stressed; (3) Emphasize high-fiber, low-glycemic-index foods, such as legumes, whole grains, nonstarchy vegetables, lean protein (tofu, cold-water fish, low-fat unsweetened dairy) eaten in small amounts, frequently throughout the day; (4) Avoid sugar, alcohol, salt, and caffeinated drinks; (5) Reduce saturated fat (from animal foods) and shift to eating more healthy, unsaturated fats, which are found in liquid vegetable oils (e.g., flaxseed oil, olive oil). *Supplements*—(1) A soluble-fiber supplement to promote fullness; (2) A probiotic supplement to heal gut tissue and support immunity and metabolism; (3) Fish oil to reduce inflammation (obesity is an inflammatory state); (4) A high-quality multivitamin and mineral for healthy metabolism and blood sugar balance; (5) Additional chromium for blood sugar balance, if needed.

Emotion(s): Insecurity, inadequacy, fear

Limiting belief(s): I am not enough. Being larger gives me more weight with others. I am not safe without my layers.

Power animal: Peacock

Flower essence(s): Angelica, Buttercup, Goldenrod, Larch, Mountain Pride, Pretty face

Affirmation(s): I am my perfect weight. My body is a divine vehicle that enables me to manifest my highest good. I am whole and complete at my innermost core.

Visualization: Find your feet on the earth. Make sure your connection with the earth is solid and strong. Breathe deeply, extracting healing energy from your union with this loving planet, letting that energy sink into the soles of your feet to fully ground you.

See yourself surrounded by people who love you. You hold hands with a circle of these dear friends. An unbroken thread of trust and support circulates through each of your hands until all of you are infused with a newfound bond. Each of you feels a strong connection in your heart center. With a gentle inhale, you extend a bow of gratitude to everyone in the circle.

You release your hands from theirs, stepping now into the circle of them. As you do, your eyes make soulful contact with each of them. You feel deeply loved for exactly who you are, and you feel a blanket of warm safety and security cover your being. Your feet tingle with this new energy, mixing with the energy of the earth.

With an inhale, you come to the realization that you have everything you need to be safe, secure, and complete. On the exhale, you release all that serves you incorrectly, releasing any residues into the ground to be transformed by the earth.

In an instant, you are presented with a large mirror, and when you peer into it, you notice you are perfectly shaped for your life's purpose. You love and appreciate every aspect of this image fully, and each member in the circle bows to this beautiful person you are. The mirror dissolves, and you are left with an inner feeling of peace.

A reset button has been pushed within your body's wiring, leaving you completely in tune with the inherent wisdom of your body. You can hear its messages about what to eat, how to move, how to live life for your highest good. Your body speaks to you freely, giving you only messages of health and wellness. And you listen intently and follow its advice, trusting its instinct. You feel whole, and perfection fills your being.

You raise your arms to the sky, like wings of a bird, and you feel free and light. Your gaze flows to the ground, and you see many layers that you have shed and no longer need at this time—old emotional hurts and wounds and depleting relationships and situations. You are free. You are light. And you enjoy your connection to your body.

Meditation: Engage in a full-length mirror meditation by focusing on your image in a mirror without judgment.

Panic Attacks

Physical description: A sudden episode of intense fear and anxiety that triggers the body to enter a fight-or-flight reaction.

Energy center(s): Root, solar plexus, heart

Nourishment: *Diet*—(1) Avoid the following: caffeine in all forms, alcohol, and refined carbohydrates; (2) Balance blood sugar with high-fiber, low-glycemic-index foods, such as legumes, whole grains, non-starchy vegetables, and fruits; (3) Eat when relaxed and try to avoid eating when stressed. *Supplements*—(1) A multivitamin and mineral supplement with special emphasis on magnesium; (2) B-complex vitamin and vitamin C for additional adrenal support; (3) Docosahexaenoic acid (DHA) from algae or fish sources.

Emotion(s): Extreme fear, fright

Limiting belief(s): I am out of here! It's not safe to be in my body. My spirit dissociates from my body. I am under attack.

Power animal: Skunk

Flower essence(s): Aspen, Garlic, Oregon Grape

Affirmation(s): I am safe and content. My body and spirit are strong, united, and free under all circumstances. My internal environment keeps calm and centered at all times.

Visualization: While in a comfortable position, preferably seated, allow your eyes to close and your hands to rest comfortably on your legs. Fix your internal gaze in the middle of your chest, in the heart area. Sit peacefully and quietly for a couple of seconds, absorbing the silence and the underlying peace embedded in every fleeting moment. Realize that in all moments, you are connected to the wisdom and vastness of the universe; in this realm, you feel supported and loved. Savor the moments of quiet until you become so still that you begin to hear the rhythm of your heart in the silence. Listen to it with the innocence of a child. Notice its purity, and let your consciousness flow with the steady beat after beat that keeps you engaged in life. Tune in even deeper to your personal rhythm, and with each beat, notice yourself traveling further into your lotuslike heart. Take as much time as you need to do so.

In your heart space rests a large lotus flower in full bloom. Its petals extend 360 degrees around, spanning your chest, armpits, and upper middle back. When you feel love, her petals expand even wider, about three feet all around you. From the lotus flower, see tendrils of white energy grounded into the center of the lotus and reaching out through every petal. A network of white energy tendrils surrounds your heart space and even the nonphysical area in front, back, and on the sides of your heart. These tendrils wind their way up into the area of your head and down into the pit of your belly. You feel safe, assured, and content in the presence of your blooming-lotus heart.

The stem of the lotus, green and strong, is felt throughout the core of your body, traveling the length of the spinal column and planted in your pelvis. With your mind's eye, you see the four strong roots of the lotus hanging down your legs, two in the left leg and two in the right leg. Her roots make their way through your feet and burrow deep into the core of the earth. Her connection to the earth gives her a feeling of stability and groundedness. These feelings ripple through your cellular consciousness. Your heart is secure in the depths of the earth, and the earth nourishes her presence. If there is any anxiety or fear in your heart, allow the lotus flower to absorb it and send it down her shaft and roots into the earth. There is no place for fear in your heart, as it feeds on love alone. The white tendrils act to keep out any fear that may try to find its way into the labyrinth of your heart lotus. When you remember the lotus in any moment that you feel insecure or unsafe, you will be protected from any feelings of panic or dread.

Let yourself sink into this beautiful connection with your heart. If you feel the need to speak words into your heart or to dialogue, take some moments now to do that. And when you have completed this exchange, put both hands on your heart area and breathe into the lotus. Feel your love circulate through your hands into the lotus, through your body, and into the earth. Give gratitude for having a heart that blossoms in love, wisdom, and beauty. And then return your hands to your sides, opening your eyes to the outer world.

Meditation: Meditate or journal on the following: (1) What do I feel that I cannot escape from? (2) What are ways that I can feel free?

Periodontitis (See Gum Disease)

Polycystic Ovarian Syndrome (See Ovarian Cysts)

Premenstrual Syndrome (PMS)

Physical description: An imbalance of hormones in a woman's body due to the onset of menstruation; may lead to emotional instability, food cravings, breast tenderness, and fatigue.

Energy center(s): Sacral, third eye

Nourishment: *Diet*—(1) Emphasize high-fiber, plant-based foods, especially soy (if you're not allergic); (2) Refrain from eating foods laden in additives, salt, refined carbohydrates, caffeine, and saturated fats; (3) Eat sources of healthy oils such as flaxseed meal and oil; cold-water fish; green, leafy vegetables; nuts; and seeds; (4) Eat small, frequent, low-glycemic-index snacks and meals throughout the day to keep blood sugar balanced; (5) Choose organically grown foods as much as possible to reduce the intake of toxic chemicals that tax the liver's detoxification system. *Supplements*—(1) A high-quality, high-potency multivitamin and mineral; (2) Additional mineral supplement if needed, with emphasis on calcium and magnesium; (3) Anti-inflammatory oil supplement from fish or flaxseed oil (fish preferred); (4) Anti-PMS botanicals, such as black cohosh, chasteberry, licorice, and dong quai.

Emotion(s): Worry, irritation, sadness, changing moods, frustration with being female, guilt regarding sexuality, tension with male figures

Limiting belief(s): My qualities as a woman are not appreciated. I feel unsafe being feminine. I am not able to express my true self as a woman for fear of being shunned. I feel conflicted about my sexuality.

Power animal: Crocodile

Flower essence(s): Alpine Lily, Basil, Easter Lily, Hibiscus, Pomegranate, Sticky Monkeyflower, Sunflower, Tiger Lily

Affirmation(s): I am fully feminine and woman in my own right. I resonate with the divine feminine nature within me, which is perfectly balanced and free. The feminine and masculine parts within me are in harmony. Sexuality is a powerful, beautiful, sacred force within me.

Visualization: See the divine feminine in you expressed as a breathtaking, gorgeous, lush tropical garden, filled with an abundance of trees, bushes, plants, food, and flowers. Imagine this landscape within the area of your low belly and hips. See the diversity of plants that inhabit this sacred space within you. The ivy that curls lovingly around your hips; the soft-petaled, melon-colored roses that infuse the garden with loving kindness; the large green leaves layered over each other providing support to one another—all life lives in harmony in this sacred space. Take a deep breath in to inhale the freshness and aliveness of this life here. Every tree you encounter bears tasty fruit—sweet, smooth mangoes; plump, sun-ripened papayas. Notice the gentle breeze in the air and all the plants swaying in a perfect rhythm.

You see a beautiful woman who tends to this garden. She visits it every day and cares for the garden by allowing it to express all of its wonderful, glorious colors and fruits. During the day, she ensures that the garden gets the right amount of sunshine, which invigorates the plant life with energy to expand and bask in the sunrays. The plants begin to dance in the vibration of this glorious yellow-orange light. At the same time, your belly expands with your breath to let the permeating sunlight to shine in, clearing away all unhappiness and infusing you with joy and peace. You feel the energy of the dazzling sunrays shine through your entire being, through each fingertip, each toe, and each strand of hair on your head. You are bathed in beauty and acceptance.

Over the course of the day, the garden becomes soaked with the golden light until it gradually shifts into darkness, making way for the moon to rise high in the sky, showing its luminescent, full face. The garden glows in the moon-filled night, enveloped in glittering, silver light, which is cooling and helps you to be creative and intuitive. At the same time you soak this light in through your fingertips, toes, and hair strands, each plant becomes nourished by its presence. With a gentle belly breath, you extend the moonlight's creative, life-giving force through every part of you.

The two streams of sunlight and moonlight come together within the garden space, swirling and dancing in harmony. You delight at their union. A ribbon of this sun-moon energy feeds each plant at its root and infuses the soil. The flowers become brighter, the fruits become riper, and the leaves extend out to all of life around it. The beautiful gardener smiles gracefully and holds out her arms in gratitude to nature. You take in her beauty, light, and balance, allowing it to penetrate every part of your physical body. You extend this brilliance to your emotional body. The two come together in perfect unison.

Meditation: Find time to connect with a community of like-minded women to create an ongoing network of support. Create a women's meditation or prayer circle.

Prostate Problems (Benign Prostatic Hyperplasia, Enlarged Prostate, Prostatitis)

Physical description: The prostate gland, an essential part of the male reproductive organs, produces an alkaline fluid for the transmission of sperm. Prostatitis is inflammation or irritation of the prostate. Benign prostatic hyperplasia (BPH) refers to enlargement of the prostate. Since the prostate gland is in close proximity to the urinary bladder, any changes in prostate function may alter urination.

Energy center(s): Root

Nourishment: *Diet*—(1) Eat an organically grown, high-protein, whole-foods diet that includes nuts, seeds (especially pumpkin), soybeans, vegetables, fruits, brown rice, cold-water fish, and legumes; (2) Avoid refined carbohydrates, caffeine, and alcohol; (3) Reduce saturated fat from animal sources and shift to healthy, unsaturated, liquid oils, such as flaxseed, olive, canola, and sesame seed; (4) For prostatitis, drink adequate fluid. *Supplements*—(1) Zinc for healthy hormone balance; (2) Flaxseed or fish oil to reduce inflammation; (3) Pumpkin-seed oil; (4) Saw palmetto; (5) Beta-sitosterol.

Emotion(s): Irritation, fear, doubts about productivity, despair, frustration with being male

Limiting belief(s): My creativity is stifled. I fear losing control. My job irritates/frustrates me.

Power animal: Ant

Flower essence(s): Indian Paintbrush, Saguaro, Tiger Lily

Affirmation(s): I am confident in my creative, masculine nature. I flow with the impulse of my creativity. I release all control and fully dive into the unfolding of life. I am one with my masculine nature. I work without limits or attachment to outcome.

Visualization: See yourself in the Mediterranean region of Europe, in the country of Italy. Envision that you are pedaling your way seamlessly through the gentle hills of Tuscany on a bicycle. The weather is warm but not hot, and the sun shines on your back, relaxing you completely from the stresses of your everyday life. You pass field after field of vineyards, olive groves, and tomato plants. There is not a care in your mind. The gentle breeze caresses your face and streams through your hair.

After awhile, you stop at a farm that grows tomatoes. The tomatoes sit comfortably on their vines, like plump, shining rubies. You decide to take a bite into a juicy tomato, and you savor its incredible, sun-kissed sweetness and soft texture. As you eat the tomato with full awareness, your body extracts from it the nutrients you need, like lycopene. And, in particular, these nutrients travel down into the base of your torso, into where your prostate gland resides. Your prostate gland feels healed by these nutrients. Any swelling or inflammation begins to subside within seconds. The energy of red from the lycopene feeds your root chakra, bringing into balance your sense of worth as a man as it is connected to your ability to survive and feel secure in the physical world. The red vibration removes any fears about making a living or how you manifest creative, masculine energy. In an instant, you feel alive and invigorated. Your confidence is restored, and your creativity in full swing.

You decide to get back on your bicycle and explore a bit further. Eventually, you end up at an olive grove with a neighboring vineyard. You are presented with fresh olives and grapes, and the farmers working in the fields offer you fresh-pressed olive oil and a glass of fine red wine. You are filled with generosity for their gifts, and you take in the energy of the oil and wine. They mix within your mouth, swirling together, and their vibration drifts down to all parts of your body, filling you with fluidity to help you release any stuck emotions. These emotions become transformed in the matrix of oil and wine into substances that can nourish your emotional body. And once again, you sense a phenomenal release of positive energy and flow in your body.

When you feel satisfied, you decide to sit under one of the olive trees in the shade. Collect all parts of your renewed self through your breath, and when you are feeling utterly relaxed yet invigorated, open your eyes and affirm, "I am confident in my creative, masculine nature."

Meditation: Find a group of men that you can connect with on a creative endeavor—such as participating in a book club, playing a team sport, or taking a woodworking or carpentry class.

Prostatitis (See Prostate Problems)

Psoriasis

Physical description: An autoimmune skin disorder characterized by skin-cell buildup, which appears as patches of scaly, reddish skin usually affecting the scalp, wrists, elbows, knees, nails, genitals, and ankles. It can also affect the joints (psoriatic arthritis).

Energy center(s): Root

Nourishment: *Diet*—(1) Work with a qualified health professional to identify food allergies; (2) Avoid inflammatory foods, such as those that are highly processed (high in sugar and trans fat), dairy, gluten, alcohol, and animal products, as much as possible; (3) Emphasize high-fiber foods, such as fruits, vegetables, whole grains, and beans; (4) Eat wild-caught salmon or, if you're vegetarian, incorporate flaxseed oil into your daily regimen; (5) Aim to eat foods in their raw state, such as raw vegetables and fruits and seeds and nuts that have been sprouted. *Supplements*—(1) To improve digestive function and eliminate toxins in the gut, use betaine hydrochloric acid for protein digestion (use under supervision of practitioner) and/or pancreatic enzymes; (2) Multivitamin containing essential nutrients for healthy skin: vitamin A, B complex, vitamin C, vitamin D, and vitamin E, along with zinc; (3) Omega-3 fatty acids in the form of fish or flaxseed oil; (4) Liver-support botanicals, such as silymarin and goldenseal.

Emotion(s): Shame, denial, anger

Limiting belief(s): I am ashamed to expose my true self. I refuse to accept my true self. I hold my anger within for fear of being hurt. My real self is sloughing away. I try to bury my shame, but it gets under my skin. I am reluctant to transform into a new me.

Power animal: Snake

Flower essence(s): Agrimony, Beech, Scleranthus

Affirmation(s): I feel secure in exposing who I truly am. I open the pores of my skin to experiencing life. I expand into transformation.

Visualization: You are walking along a path on a warm summer day in a forest, and although the sun is shining, you feel cool relief from the shade spotting your path. Your skin is open and receptive to the temperature of the environment. Your skin is your body's landscape of the senses. Through your skin, you receive so much information about your interaction with your outer world.

Stop from proceeding forward on this path and find yourself a small tree. You make your way over to a beautiful, aromatic cedar tree and sit down under it, with your spine against the body of the tree. You can feel its strength and gather insight from touching its skin, its bark. With your eyes closed, you let your skin do the observing around you, feeling the comfortable grass beneath you, the breeze through your fingertips and caressing your scalp. You feel at one with this moment and with the fullness of who you are.

Across from you, you notice a small hot spring. Your skin calls out for you to take a dip and nourish it with these healing waters. You walk over to the spring, shed your clothes, and slowly slip into the comfortably warm, bubbling water. The smell of sulfur casually wafts through the air. You are aware of the healing nature of sulfur for the skin. On the count of three—one, two, three—you immerse your entire body into the water. You hold your breath for a count of three underneath the water—one, two, three—and when you come up, you instantly feel pure and fresh, full of energy. This healing water soothes your skin, relieving any inflammation, and helps your skin to renew itself immediately.

Looking down and around at the skin on your body, you see these changes unfold before you. Any scaling, red skin has been replaced with a new layer of vibrant skin. You are overjoyed at the transformation. And as this is happening, you begin to get insight as to what might be "getting under your skin" or what has been irritating you lately. You may even begin to see images of people, places, or situations that have been trapped within your external boundary—your skin. Envision them releasing from you as new skin layers your body surface. See solutions for them with the help of your fresh, renewed skin. Listen to any insight your new skin has to offer for the subtle and not-so-subtle irritations in your life that inflame you.

With a deep breath, let your body sink into the magical springwater again. Feel the bubbles from underneath, tickling your feet. And as you emerge from the water another time, let yourself be wrapped in a feeling of playfulness. You have the ability to shake off anything that finds its way "under your skin" by going with the flow of life and by releasing tight control on your life. Invite your self to soak in the spring for as long as you desire. *(Pause here for a couple of seconds or minutes.)*

When you are ready to go on your way, carefully climb out of the spring. Let all the nourishing spring droplets dotting your body soak themselves in to your skin. After this cleansing, purifying, and soaking process, your skin is simply radiant. It has a shine and glow that all will notice and identify as healthy, well-cared-for skin.

You get dressed and walk back to the cedar tree. This time, instead of having your back to the cedar tree, you face it directly, holding its trunk with your outstretched arms. The cedar tree, which loves you so much, infuses you with its green energy of nature, which seals in your healing from the springwater. The green energy saturates your skin entirely, making its way into every pore, smoothing out all wrinkles. Once your skin has drunk in the energy of the cedar tree, you feel that, at a deep level, you have taken in an elixir of love and forgiveness. And with these gifts, you express your gratitude, bow your head, and turn to walk toward your path—your path of life.

Meditation: Imagine your skin laid out like a large mat before you. Meditate on its smoothness, calmness, and perfection. When you feel a sense of loving kindness towards your skin, see it transform to a healing robe that cloaks your soul. Sit in silence, feeling its acceptance and warmth.

Rheumatoid Arthritis

Physical description: An autoimmune condition involving chronic inflammation of the synovial membrane surrounding the joints; can ultimately cause joint destruction, loss of function, and deformity.

Energy center(s): Root

Nourishment: *Diet*—(1) Work with a qualified healthcare professional to identify food allergies using an elimination diet (food allergies result in an imbalanced immune system); (2) Emphasize whole foods, such as vegetables, legumes, whole grains (no gluten), and fruits, and try to make a majority of your intake the raw or sprouted forms of these foods; (3) Remove animal products from the diet (especially fatty meats and dairy) except for fish; (4) Focus on high omega-3 foods, such as flaxseed oil; green, leafy vegetables; nuts; seeds; and fish. *Supplements*—(1) Omega-3 fats in the form of fish or flaxseed oil; (2) Support digestion with betaine hydrochloric acid (for protein digestion; caution: consult practitioner on how to use) and pancreatic enzymes. Both supplements can be taken with meals. Pancreatic enzymes can be taken in between meals to reduce inflammation; (3) A complete multivitamin containing vitamins C and E and zinc; (4) Probiotic supplement to reestablish healthy gut flora; (5) Anti-inflammatory botanicals, such as curcumin, ginger, bromelain, and quercetin.

Emotion(s): Resentment and anger towards self and others

Limiting belief(s): Other people have done things to me that I am angry about. I despise myself for holding back.

Power animal: Raccoon

Flower essence(s): Willow, Goldenrod

Affirmation(s): I am open to receiving and giving in equal measure. I move through life like a cool, flowing stream of water. I release. I let go of pain. I accept all parts of myself.

Visualization: Imagine you have been invited into a special healing room. You open the door to enter, and immediately your nostrils are filled with the aroma of lavender. You breathe in the subtle lavender smell, and it pervades your being with a soft wisdom and feeling of relaxation.

In the room, you see a table for you to lie on. The rest of the room is relatively free of any distraction. There is no noise, and there are no images or objects other than the table. You are guided to lie down on the table, and as you do, you have the feeling that you are sinking into a warm feather bed. Your entire body is cushioned by the table, and because you feel such trust and support, you decide to let your body go completely, making it heavy, like sandbags. The bottom layer of you, closest to the table, sinks in a bit further, and the other layers resting above start to collapse towards the table, one right after another. Your body feels like it is descending downwards, and, indeed, it is. The table is slowly transporting you down below the ground in a very gradual, safe manner. The entire time, you are warm and comfortable, and the lavender scent continues to ribbon around your being.

After descending about twenty feet, the table stops, and you look around you, noticing that you have entered a cave filled wall to wall with diamonds and amethyst gems. There is so much radiance and vibration within this space that you become overwhelmed with bliss. The diamond energy sparkles forth like little stars, illuminating the room and especially your body. Any inflammation you feel in your joints or that is lingering in any tissue, organ, or cell, is drawn out from you like a magnet by the diamond stars. In place of the inflammation, you are penetrated, from 360 degrees, by the brilliance of the diamond light, which brings peace and love to you. Take a couple of moments to soak in this white diamond bath of light, ridding your body of all excess that makes you imbalanced and gives you symptoms. Breathe in the lavender-scented air. Feel your body completely cushioned and free from any pain. Right now, every cell in your body shines with the essence of the diamond energy, which brings to you not material wealth, but abundant self-worth beyond measure. You feel alert, alive, and centered on the present moment. Your conscious awareness is as expansive as the nighttime sky, glittering with its own diamond stars.

As you pull yourself back into the cavern of diamond and amethyst, you now begin to notice the multifaceted amethyst clusters and geodes that line the cave. You look at them intently, as their energy is mesmerizing and miraculous. As you continue to gaze, you observe that they are moving towards you—not the amethyst alone, but also an angel holding each amethyst. These angels, bearing amethysts, walk towards you in a loving way, assembling around your body and surrounding you with the protective, cleansing energy of amethyst in addition to the grace and radiance of each angel. Amethysts are placed over your main seven chakras as well as your forty-two minor chakras. Your being basks in the purple glow of amethyst and the healing love of angels. Absorb this energy, and use it to help shift your body, emotions, and mind into a higher state of awareness. Allow it to help you shed past ideas that no longer serve you. Let it connect you with your highest self. Through the vision of amethyst, see yourself in your most healthy, radiant, beautiful, and true form ever. And you become that form, with the help of your breath. Breathe in amethyst energy and watch it intermingle with the spiraled DNA in each cell of your being. At a deep level, you feel whole, relaxed, and nourished by the essence of who you are.

When you feel that this exercise has completed, let your heart swell with gratitude for the diamonds, amethysts, and angels. Offer to them your thanks. The table begins to glide upwards, and after a couple of seconds, you find yourself back in the healing room. You rise up and stretch your body, noticing that your joints feel free of any pain or inflammation. You walk out of the doorway and looking behind you, you observe that the healing room has disappeared.

Meditation: Meditate in the presence of a piece of amethyst. As you focus on your breath, allow your joint stiffness, pain, and/or swelling to be directed outward, at the amethyst. Let the precious stone absorb what you no longer need, transforming it. Then imagine that your joints are bathed in purple, healing energy. Spend most of your meditation time basking in the amethyst glow.

Right-Side-of-Body Complaints

Physical description: The right side of the body corresponds to the masculine (yang) part of our nature—that which is direct, linear, logical, and secure in the physical world. A greater proportion of symptoms on the right side of the body would indicate that there is an imbalance in that quality of one's life.

Energy center(s): Root, solar plexus, throat

Nourishment: Protein is the nutrient with the most masculine resonance, as it is the builder of body tissues and oversees a multitude of functions in the body. If you are deficient in masculine energy, eating more protein (particularly animal protein, if you are not vegetarian) may be harmonizing. Conversely, if there is too much masculine energy, reducing protein or shifting to vegetarian protein sources may be of benefit.

Emotion(s): Aggression (if masculine energy is excessive) or insecurity (if masculine energy is deficient)

Limiting belief(s): Challenges with authority and father figures. *If masculine energy is excessive:* I'll control others before they will control me. *If masculine energy is deficient:* I give up my power.

Power animal: Bull

Flower essence(s): Holly, Larkspur (if excessive); Mountain Pride (if deficient)

Affirmation(s): The masculine part of my nature is balanced. I am in harmony. The yin and yang within me are in equal measure. I am confident and strong. I have a healthy sense of authority and leadership.

Visualization: Close your eyes. Take a breath. On your next breath, move your awareness down to the space right below your feet. See yourself grounded, firmly planted into the earth. With your next inhale, see your breath rising in from below your feet and moving up into your legs. Have the essence of the breath distill into your low back. Repeat the breath movement again, pulling it up from the solid earth foundation and into your legs, and letting it find its way into your tailbone area once again. Allow yourself to indulge in the movement of your breath through your legs a few more times, and with each time, you feel more and more at peace, relaxed, ready to explore the right side of your body.

Once you feel a sense of calm pervade you, take a moment to do a body scan of the right side of your body, starting with your head and moving slowly down to your toes. Note any areas that call out to you and observe what they are trying to say. Be the mindful observer as you scan, not having any judgments, opinions, or thoughts about what is being revealed to you. The more observant you are, the more will be unveiled to you. Take your time; be patient with the process.

Notice any places that appear to not be moving with the flow of your breath and with the river of your blood. Go deeper into these places, using your breath. Breathe into them, one by one, receiving any information they are willing to impart. Once you have arrived at your feet, take a deep breath, carrying the energy of earth up into your low back, returning your energy to your feet with the exhale. Take a moment to ask yourself, "Where do I need to show more of my warrior energy in my life?" Let your answer come forth. And then proceed to ask, "Where does my life need movement?" Wait for your answer from the right side of your body. Examine whether there are within you any issues about letting go of your ability to lead your life. How do you lead yourself in your daily life, and how do you impact others with your leadership?

Continue to breathe, directing your breath into the right side of the body, giving it the support it needs to fully unfold. Observe the answers coming through, resting them inside the chambers of your heart so you can come back to them and reflect on them more deeply at another time.

Once you are satisfied that you have enough answers to work with and decipher, let your mind's eye create an image of your internal warrior. Imagine qualities of yourself in this warrior—strength, authority, the power of presence and action. See them encompassed in the aura of this warrior part of you. Let yourself dialogue with your warrior. What do you want to say to these parts of yourself? What do you need to listen to from this archetype? Direct any and all wisdom into your heart area for further contemplation.

Beyond your warrior image, see the line of your male ancestors— your father, grandfather, great-grandfather, great-great-grandfather— going back several hundreds of generations. See the essence of the warrior archetype like a glowing thread within all of your male ancestors, holding the family lineage, until it finally connects to your warrior image. Envision this connection strengthening and, at the same time, balancing your masculine qualities with your female qualities. Breathe in this strength and balance through your connection to the earth, and let go of any deficiency or imbalance through the soles of your feet. Give thanks to your male ancestors for their contribution to you. As you do so, their images slowly fade away until you are left with your warrior image. At this moment, you feel welcomed to step into your warrior image so it becomes you and balances you, particularly the right side of your body. In an instant, you feel whole and complete.

Allow yourself to slowly open your eyes. You feel grounded, balanced, and supported. When you feel ready, let yourself enter into the cavern of your heart to explore any messages you may have received from the right side of your body, and journal your responses.

Meditation: Engage your warrior nature in meditative writing. Let this part of you write, without being controlled or censored, for five minutes per day.

Sciatica

Physical description: Sciatica refers to leg pain, numbness, weakness, or tingling felt in the low back, buttock, and/or parts of the leg and feet due to compression of a nerve in the lower half of the body, such as lumbar, sacral, and sciatic nerves.

Energy center(s): Root, crown

Nourishment: *Diet*—(1) Focus on anti-inflammatory foods, such as whole, raw, fresh foods (vegetables, fruits), and reduce inflammatory foods, such as fried foods, fatty red meat, sugar, and hydrogenated oils; (2) Drink adequate water to help keep muscles hydrated. *Supplements*—(1) B-complex vitamin (especially vitamins B1 and B6, which are important in nerve health); (2) Calcium-magnesium supplement for healthy muscles and nerves; (3) Supplements containing anti-inflammatories, such as bromelain, quercetin, papain, boswellia, and ginger, may be helpful in reducing inflammation around nerves.

Emotion(s): Fear and doubt about survival in the physical world and about the future

Limiting belief(s): Surviving is painful. I am limited by money and my possessions. It pains me to be in my body.

Power animal: Porcupine

Flower essence(s): California Poppy

Affirmation(s): I am capable. I move forward with ease. I am eternally abundant.

Visualization: Visualize your body as a house and your nervous system as the electrical wiring inside. As though you were your body's expert electrician, put your awareness in a tiny vehicle and start to course through the network of nerves in your body. Healthy nerves are signals firing back and forth to one another in the perfect rhythm and amplitude. Note whether you see any unhealthy transmissions between nerves that can lead to poor function or pain. In particular, draw your focus to the area of your low back, buttocks, and legs. Observe whether you see any strain on your electrical system, whether the nerves are being impinged upon or are out of place, and if you see this, use your special tools to get into the space to correct the situation, making sure the nerves are free and the electricity is flowing.

You have some unhealthy nerve activity in this area of your body that is causing you pain. See this pain in your body manifest like strong lightning rods in the sky—unpredictable, sharp, shooting pain that radiates through you. The electricity in your body is chaotic and unbalanced in this area. The next time you feel or see this pain happening, visualize these lightning rods of current moving through your legs, into your feet, and grounding the energy deep into the layers of the earth. Keep your legs apart, unrestricted, and let the electrical, sharp, shooting pain run through you and ground, so it can dissipate its energy rather than continue to reoccur in your body. Each time you feel the pain, direct it far away from your body, several feet into the ground.

As part of the final repair of your nervous/electrical system, run through your body a fresh current of white light, starting at the top of your head, moving through your brain, through your eyes, and into every nerve network and bundle in your body. This white light imparts the ability of your nerves to transmit smoothly and evenly, and corrects any other imbalance.

When you feel ready, remove your consciousness from your vehicle, and magnify yourself into the present moment.

Meditation: Meditate on the network of your nervous system. In your mind's eye, focus on streaming calm pulses with your breath through your nerve bundles.

Sexually Transmitted Disease (See Venereal Disease)

Sinus Congestion

Physical description: Inflammation of the sinuses and nasal passages due to viral or bacterial infection or allergies, which results in thick mucus accumulation in or discharge from the nose, as well as swelling and pressure in the eyes, nose, cheeks, and head.

Energy center(s): Throat, third eye

Nourishment: *Diet*—(1) Work with a qualified healthcare professional to identify food allergies; (2) Avoid sugar-containing foods and dairy in all forms. *Supplements*—(1) Vitamin C and bioflavonoids for immune support; (2) Bromelain (a pineapple-derived enzyme) taken between meals; (3) Quercetin for anti-inflammatory activity.

Emotion(s): Hurt, grief

Limiting belief(s): I hold back. My life feels like it's moving too slowly and painfully. My grief accumulates. I feel pressured.

Power animal: Pig

Flower essence(s): Mustard, Walnut, Yerba Santa

Affirmation(s): I forgive. I release all barriers to my personal growth. I breathe in fresh life-force energy and release all that blocks me. I am open to life.

Visualization: Close your eyes and open your vision to a new landscape—the expanse of the ocean before you. The sun sits high in the sky, and its rays are captured within the tiny droplets that spray from each wave coming in to shore. See yourself on the brink of the ocean, and your feet washed over by the water with each incoming wave of breath. Extend your arms to both sides to absorb the wonderful salty air.

On your next inhale, breathe in the mist arising from this great, purifying body of water. The mist sprays the internal circuit of your nasal passages, tickling them with its presence. You breathe in its essence fully and deeply, and then you relax and exhale gently. And with the rise of the next ocean wave, you inhale, and with the receding of the wave towards the shore, you exhale. You spend a full minute allowing your breathing to parallel the movement of the ocean, and the whole time you are being permeated by the droplets of its essence, which are dispersed through the air in the process. Inhaling and exhaling, inhaling and exhaling, you feel that you become the ocean waters. You merge with the expanse of this greatness, and its healing energy ripples through your body.

As the waves of healing move through you, your own breath unified with that of the ocean, you begin releasing all the congestion that has been blocking you from movement in your own life. Those blocks all seem so small, and they dissolve with the movement of your breath. They are liberated from you, tossed into the voluminous ocean depths to be torn apart and regenerated into more healing water droplets. Your sinus passages, which curl like conch shells throughout the middle to upper part of your face and forehead, are especially clear of any debris or stagnation. They have been opened more fully as you breathe in the ocean-cleansed air. This air has purified the entire nasal cavity, enabling you to breathe the eternal life-force energy deeply and fully in the moment. With each breath, you feel more equipped to accept and embrace the events that life sends your way like ocean waves. Any time you feel overwhelmed, you can return to the healing ocean setting and ask to be cleansed by the saltwater.

And now gather up your arms to your chest, taking the purity of the ocean waves into every cell of your being. Wiggle your toes in the water that meets your feet, and open your eyes to the expanse of your new life.

Meditation: Engage in a simple meditation in which you observe the journey of your inhale and exhale through your nasal passages. Observe where there is resistance.

Skin Irritation (See Hives, Itching, Psoriasis)

Stomach Problems (See Heartburn, Indigestion, Stomach Ulcers)

Stomach Ulcers

Physical description: A painful lesion or erosion in the mucosal lining of the digestive tract. (If in the stomach, called a stomach or gastric ulcer; if in the upper small intestine, a duodenal ulcer.)

Energy center(s): Solar plexus

Nourishment: *Diet*—(1) Identify food allergies with the help of a qualified healthcare practitioner; (2) Avoid common food sources that can irritate the stomach, such as coffee, alcohol, acidic fruits (e.g., oranges, lemons, grapefruit), and spicy foods; (3) Eat smaller meals more frequently throughout the day; (4) Increase consumption of high-fiber foods, like beans and vegetables; (5) For fluids, try fresh cabbage juice, aloe vera juice, and peppermint and chamomile teas. *Supplements*—(1) Multivitamin containing vitamins A, C, and zinc to help promote healthy gut lining; (2) Deglycyrrhizinated licorice (or DGL, a form of licorice without a compound that normally causes high blood pressure).

Emotion(s): Worry

Limiting belief(s): I can't take it all in. I try to digest my life, but it is overwhelming. Worry consumes me.

Power animal: Cow (ruminants have multiple stomachs!)

Flower essence(s): Cherry Plum, Dogwood

Affirmation(s): I transform all life experiences into information I can use. I process my life with mindfulness, ease, and love. I can stomach all that comes my way.

Visualization: Close your eyes and place your right hand on the middle of your torso, right underneath your ribs. Place your left hand on top of your right hand. As you breathe in, focus your awareness on the area where your hands lay—the central point of your stomach. Bring your breath to this area repeatedly. Feel the accumulation of the energy of the breath within the reservoir of your stomach.

See your stomach as a place to receive. All the food we bring to our stomachs is like an offering to our bodies. See your stomach as a crucible, bringing forth the element of fire within the body to begin the process of transformation. Sometimes we deliver to our stomachs more than food; we feed it with stress, causing it to become tight. With your next inhale, see your stomach relaxing its wall. Let the breath melt away any tension in the stomach. Breathe in peace, and breathe out tightness. Breathe in acceptance, and breathe out expectations.

Imagine that before you rests a vial of golden, liquid syrup containing protective energy for your stomach. In your mind's eye, place your hands on the vial, and focus on your infinite, seamless ability to process and break down life and to absorb the lessons you are given. Infuse into this glistening, warm liquid the gifts of transformation and personal power. Bring the vial to your lips, swallowing the smooth, flowing, honeylike liquid of protection, transformation, and empowerment. See it travel slowly down your throat and coat the lining of your esophagus. You feel a pleasant, inner sensation of peace. And with your breath, you guide the liquid down into your stomach, like an offering placed on the sacred altar of your body. This liquid is what you need at this moment to repair any damage to your stomach. See it coating the inner stomach, penetrating and healing any ulcerations of the lining. Notice how it brings into balance the stomach-acid levels and washes away any residual effects of stress. Your stomach feels nourished and soft, healed and healthy, able to make the right amount of stomach acid for your body.

Move your hands in a circular motion around your stomach, energetically receiving and disseminating the healing energy to the surrounding digestive organs. Breathe in the energy of peace. Remove your hands from your abdomen, and open your eyes slowly.

Meditation: Meditate on the area associated with your stomach. Envision it as a bag full of undigested life events—relationships, work, family, financial stress, and all other sources of worry that have come into your life. Unpack each one and meditatively reflect on it, neutrally, without worry and stress.

Stress

Physical description: The negative physical and psychological effect(s) of unhealthy stressors in the environment. Prolonged stress can lead to the development of serious diseases.

Energy center(s): Root, sacral, solar plexus, heart, throat, third eye, crown

Nourishment: *Diet*—(1) Remove "stressful" foods such as those that are low on nutrients, like highly processed, convenience foods (soft drinks; fast food; high-fat, high-sugar snack foods), caffeine, and alcohol; (2) Eat more nutrient-dense foods, such as fresh vegetables and fruits high in vitamin C. *Supplements*—(1) B-complex vitamin (ensure that adequate vitamin B5, vitamin B6, and biotin are included); (2) Vitamin C for supporting the immune system.

Emotion(s): Fear

Limiting belief(s): I am out of control. I am inadequate. No one values what I have to offer. I have to prove my worth through my accomplishments.

Power animal: Elk

Flower essence(s): Dill, Elm

Affirmation(s): I have fun in all that I do. I enjoy life. I am full and complete from within.

Visualization: Close your eyes and find yourself in a comfortable seated position. Breathe in, and use the breath to relax your muscles. Allow yourself to let go in these next few minutes and to sail within the ocean of your imagination.

With your mind's eye, see yourself in an open field full of electric green grass. The sky above you is free from any trace of a cloud, and in the distance, much to your surprise, you see a marvelous rainbow stretching through the sky. You can't help but walk towards the rainbow as it draws you in. In a few moments, you have reached the rainbow's edge.

Your instinct is to walk into the band of red color. At once, you feel a sense of safety and trust. Any fears about money or survival are shed from your body like clothing falling to the ground. You breathe in the essence of the deep, grounding red color, and in so doing, you see the roots of your being connected to the vast core of the earth. You come to an appreciation of your body's wisdom, and in honor of your body, you let go of any stress, tension, or hardness that you hold in it as a result of your daily living. The red color fills your being, giving you the strength you need to feel strong and capable to withstand any challenges you may encounter day-to-day.

You bathe in the red light for a couple more seconds before moving on to the intensely vibrant orange band of light radiating from the rainbow. The dancing orange molecules of light permeate your being, filling you with laughter and a sense of pleasure and play. At once, you feel the spirit of your childlike self surfacing. All worries are dispelled from your emotional body and replaced with contentment. You can now go with the flow of living in a way that you hadn't been able to before.

Once you've taken in as much healing orange light as you can, you take a few steps over and walk into the radiant, glistening beam of streaming yellow light. The light is so bright and sunny; it carries the possibility of power and energy that you haven't felt in a long time. Basking in its radiance sheds any feeling of being overwhelmed. In your mind's eye, you are presented with a representative movie of a typical day in your life, and you begin to see where you can better improve your management of time, your relationships with people, and even the efficiencies of your living situation. Being in the glow of yellow infuses you with a confidence that enables you to forge ahead into the unknown without the baggage of stress.

At your own pace, you transition yourself into the peaceful hue of emerald green that is next to the sunny yellow strip. The green color blankets you, almost like the towering embrace from a comforting forest. You immediately feel love and warmth entering your heart. Any stress that you had previously put on your heart is now coming undone, unwinding itself from the chamber of your heart and from the extensions of blood vessels networking through your body. This release allows you to sink into the moment even more than before. There is no more heaviness in your heart now; it is full with only the green light of nature.

From green, you walk into an aquamarine color, which has energy resembling that of the sky. You feel a sense of freedom from any restriction that may have centered around your spoken words to others. You know that all of your verbal exchanges with others will be good, true, and beautiful. No more stress blocks your true nature and expression.

When you are ready, you walk into the vibrant energy of violet, which stimulates your intuition and imagination. You realize that you have not been as attentive to your intuitive voice as you may need to be and that by listening to it, you are tapping into deep wisdom and insight about life. By connecting with violet and with your intuition, you allow yourself the gift of inner knowing, so you can make choices that benefit your highest self.

And finally, when you are saturated with the depth of violet, you can walk into the dazzling white light at the end of the rainbow. This light purifies and clears any residual stress in your being, whether that stress is in your physical, emotional, mental, or spiritual bodies. You feel at one with all your layers—perfect, whole and complete, ready to take on life's challenges and opportunities in the spirit of growth and learning.

Stepping out of the white light, you notice you have captured each of these colors within you so they are always working with you to reduce stress in your life and guide you to your higher path. On the count of seven, you will open your eyes to your new, enlightened, invigorated self.

One. Two. Three. Four. Five. Six. Seven.

Open your eyes and take a deep breath in to welcome your new state of being!

Meditation: Use laughter as a form of meditation. Allow yourself to laugh for at least one minute daily.

Stuttering

Physical description: A speaking disorder in which speech is disrupted by involuntary insertions, repetitions, or prolongations of sounds or words, making it difficult to communicate.

Energy center(s): Throat

Nourishment: Focus on how you eat. Note if your eating is erratic, quick, and mindless, and whether you rush yourself through the process. Practice taking slow, mindful bites of food, mirroring how, when speaking, you would speak in a measured, unrushed manner.

Emotion(s): Shame, fear

Limiting belief(s): I am not worthy. I am fearful of expressing myself, as there may be consequences. I lack valuable opinions, beliefs, and thoughts.

Power animal: Moose

Flower essence(s): Larch, Buttercup, Trumpet Vine

Affirmation(s): I am confident. I express my true thoughts and feelings.

Visualization: Close your eyes, relax your body, and find your way into the present moment. Focus on the space that spans your throat to your mouth; put all of your awareness here now. Feel the power and the authority of the energy that comes from the voice. Clear away any obstruction in this area by envisioning a tube of aquamarine light circled around your mouth to throat area.

This light is a repository, a place into which any areas in your mouth and voice-producing anatomy can release any blocks or lodged, old, stuck communication. Allow this sea green light into your mouth, letting it permeate your inner mouth. Swish it around your mouth like mouthwash, so it collects any energetic debris. In your mind's eye, visualize yourself expelling it from your mouth. When you do, you see in the light images or words, which provide you with insight as to why you may not have fluidity and flow in your voice and speaking. What do these trapped words and images say to you? What do you say back to them?

Now sip in more of the aquamarine light, and let it sink into the back of your throat and coat your voicebox. This coating serves as protection for preserving your truth when you speak, and it will allow you to speak without fear of making mistakes or saying something that you think may offend someone. You release fear from your truth and authenticity, releasing it from the inside and into the blue light that circles outside your throat area.

Every time the blue light receives a block or whatever stands in the way of your communication, it becomes brighter and brighter blue. When you have completed clearing your throat and voice, the blue light condenses to form a small star shape in the middle of your throat. This symbolic placement will remind you of your ability to shine forth your wisdom with words that flow forth seamlessly. From this star, all of your words are strung together, like pearls on a necklace, before they are delivered to the outside. Every message from you is heard in a perfect way, and through your complete communication, you feel that you express yourself creatively. Take a deep breath in, letting this breath rest for a second in the blue star. Every time you breathe, you cleanse the star and keep it shining bright.

When you feel it's time, gently open your eyes. Let the sound *ah* be felt in your blue star and materialize in the stream of your voice. Keep in mind that the throat is the birth canal of the heart's passions and wishes; the *ah* sound will connect your voice to that of your heart.

Meditation: Meditate using sound by chanting a vowel sound like *ah*. To do this, breathe in deeply, and on the exhale, release the *ah*.

Syphilis (See Venereal Disease)

TMJ (See Jaw Tightness)

Tooth Pain

Physical description: Tooth pain results when the nerve root of a tooth is irritated due to an infection, cavity, injury, cracked tooth, receding gums, or jaw muscle spasm, to name a few.

Energy center(s): Throat

Nourishment: *Diet*—(1) Often, tooth pain is aggravated by chewing or by extreme temperatures. Reduce the need for chewing by having more soups, sauces, and smoothies. Avoid foods that are excessively hot or cold and aim for room temperature foods; (2) Reduce foods that promote inflammation, such as fatty meats (especially processed meats or overly cooked meat), hydrogenated oils, and sugar-sweetened foods (soft drinks, juices, cakes, cookies); (3) Emphasize anti-inflammatory foods rich in omega-3 fats such as fish; flaxseed oil; green, leafy vegetables; and nuts and seeds. *Supplements*—(1) Vitamin C and bioflavonoids for healthy gum tissue; (2) Coenzyme Q10; (3) Herbal anti-inflammatories, such as those containing white willow bark, turmeric, quercetin, and ginger; (4) Herbal antibacterial supplements like neem, goldenseal, cinnamon, eucalyptus, and garlic.

Emotion(s): Anger (unexpressed), inflammation

Limiting belief(s): I hold back my angry words because of fear. My root beliefs cause me pain. It is painful to bite into life.

Power animal: Horse

Flower essence(s): Deerbrush

Affirmation(s): I speak my true feelings. I communicate my authentic self.

Visualization: Close your eyes and focus your awareness on the tooth or teeth that are causing you pain. And now dive into the pain completely by sitting with it and inviting it to be fully felt and heard. As you do this, make sure to breathe deeply and at a comfortable rate. The pounding, throbbing pain—what does it want to say to you? Give it your full attention. What sign, information, or gift is your body trying to impart to you through this pain? Where do you have pain in your life? What needs noticing? What is difficult to process? Let your inner self reflect on these answers. Let your pain speak to you.

When you feel that you have listened adequately and garnered some important information for you to reflect and journal on later, imagine you see a translucent golden sphere of energy in your throat. The sphere rotates, shining its brilliance in the confines of your throat. It extends its beams out, and one beam is directed at the root of each tooth in your mouth. Imagine that this golden energy source feeds each tooth root, pumping each one with vital energy, and at the same time, anything that needs to be released from the tooth through the root travels into the golden beam of light and back to the sphere. This exchange of energy happens simultaneously for each tooth. All remaining pain or infection is dissolved by the dazzling light of gold.

When the process has completed, draw the energy back into the sphere residing in your throat-chakra area. Bring your attention back to your mouth, to your teeth. Drink in the affirmation, "I listen to the messages of my body with attentiveness," allowing it to swirl within your mouth before you swallow it.

Meditation: Using meditation as a vehicle, dive deep into the pain in your tooth or teeth. Allow the pain to pulse its message through a silent space of meditation, so it is heard. Without judgment, let it express itself. When you have completed your meditation, log your impressions in a journal for further reflection.

Toxin Overload

Physical description: Over time, toxins accumulate in the body and gradually impair body organs and their functions. The results manifest as a variety of symptoms, ranging from fatigue and headaches to allergic reactions and memory loss. These toxins may be generated internally through the body's metabolic processes (e.g., cellular debris, free radicals, excess acid formation) or by microorganisms that may be present in the body and that manufacture their own toxic substances. Also, the body may take in toxins through its exposure to certain elements in the environment, such as polluted air, contaminated water, and foods laden with pesticides, insecticides, and herbicides.

Energy center(s): Root, sacral, solar plexus, heart, throat, third eye

Nourishment: *Diet*—(1) To reduce toxin intake, eat organically grown foods (especially free-range, organically fed animal products, if you are not vegetarian) as much as possible; (2) Drink adequate amounts of pure, filtered water (about eight 8-ounce glasses daily) to encourage toxin removal through the kidneys; (3) Consume high-fiber foods, such as legumes, whole grains, and vegetables, as fiber assists in trapping toxins in the gut and carrying them out of the body; (4) Work with a healthcare practitioner to identify food allergies; (5) Cease eating foods high in refined sugars and hydrogenated oils; (6) Eat cruciferous vegetables, such as broccoli, brussels sprouts, and cabbage, as well as high-sulfur foods, like garlic, onions, and legumes. *Supplements*—(1) Powdered-fiber supplement (e.g., psyllium, apple pectin) to enhance removal of toxins through the gut; (2) Multivitamin (that includes the B complex, vitamin C, and choline) to ensure that the liver has the nutrients it needs for effective toxin removal.

Emotion(s): Toxic emotions add to the body's toxic burden. Start tracking your emotions on a daily basis and focus specifically on those that are positive, so they become magnified (see Appendix E). If you begin a cleansing process, keep a journal to track emotional release. Anger is typically associated with the liver. Since the liver is an essential organ of cleansing, you may notice some issues around anger arising as you go through the process.

Limiting belief(s): Life is burdensome and toxic. I am invaded and overwhelmed. I find it difficult to let go.

Power animal: Frog

Flower essence(s): Angel's Trumpet, Hornbeam

Affirmation(s): I am clean. I release myself of all that serves me incorrectly. Purity pervades me.

Visualization: Close your eyes and find your breath. Once you have grounded yourself through your breathing pattern, begin exploring the landscape of your body. See your body as a vessel, a container, like a glass. Look through all places in the body to see whether you have stored excessive toxins.

Check your lungs to see what the air you breathe has brought in. Do you see darkness, discoloration, or other potential indicators of a toxin accumulation? If so, take a deep breath in, imagining that you are breathing in cleansing, purifying white light. Fill your lungs with the dazzling white-light molecules and watch how they make toxins transform into molecules of oxygen. Spend as much time as you need to ensure that your lungs are completely clean and clear.

Once your lungs are glowing with healing white light and there is no trace of any air pollutants, move your awareness to one of the main organs helping your body to detoxify—your liver, which rests in the right upper quadrant of your abdomen. Scan your liver with your mind's eye to examine whether your liver is able to remove toxins efficiently. Observe whether the liver's machinery is jammed or inactive. With your breath, visualize directing green energy of movement into your liver. This emerald green energy lubricates the machinery of the liver to make it work effectively once again. Any accumulated toxins have been pushed through and sent out of your body with the help of the nourishing green energy.

Once you feel satisfied that you have released any stuck pathways in the liver, move your attention slowly down from your liver and into the gut terrain. The intestines are several feet long and can trap harmful microorganisms, as well as toxins from our food supply. Take a deep breath of pink light, and pull it down into your small intestine. Have the pink light wind through your small intestine. Like a net, it gathers any harmful fungi, bacteria, or viruses, in addition to any compounds from food that are not beneficial for the body. Let the pink light go steadily through the long tunnel of your small intestine, and then let it enter your large intestine, where it gathers up any toxins that are excessive. Allow the pink light to exit and travel down to the earth, releasing its contents fully and completely to the planet, so they can be transformed into rejuvenative life energy to feed the forces of nature.

When you feel that your intestines are clear, travel to the back of your body to meet your kidneys, which sit on either side in the low-back region. The kidneys help to purify the water element in your body. If we do not drink enough water, the kidneys can be taxed. If we eat foods that are too high in salt or in protein, our kidneys may need to take additional action. With your breath, imagine a cool blue, watery wave working its way through your body from head to toe, cleansing all the water held in your body. Spiral this blue water around both of your kidneys simultaneously, moving from the outside of the kidney into the inside and flushing through the kidney tubules. See this water swishing through your bladder, clearing it from any micro-organisms that are unhealthy. Allow this water to exit your body by watching the streams travel down your legs and through your feet. Let all of the toxins pour out of your body through your feet and soak the earth beneath you. You feel entirely cleansed and pure.

The last organ is your largest organ of detoxification—the covering of your body, your skin. Think of all the contact that your skin has with the environment and how it can easily accumulate and absorb toxins, whether through water, air, or personal-care products. Our skin equips us with the large surface area and multitude of openings, or pores, which are needed to excrete toxins. With your last deep breath, breathe in a soft yellow light and allow it to penetrate your entire skin, shining its light through the thousands of pores.

When you are satisfied with the penetration of the yellow light through your skin, allow yourself to take a couple of minutes to bask in your new glow of health and purity. Scan your body one more time, seeing the result of the clearing done by all the different lights—the white light in the lungs, green light in the liver, pink light in the intestines, blue light in the kidneys, and yellow light in the skin. Let all of these colorful lights coalesce in the center of your torso. Cup your hands and fill them with the swirling mixture of this light. Expand your hands out all around you, forming a protective colorful shield of light.

In your own time, gently open your eyes. Notice the feeling of energy and clarity that you have. Give yourself thanks for this beautiful cleansing!

Meditation: Meditate while basking in sunlight or while imagining that you are engulfed by a glow of purifying white light.

Urinary Tract Infection (Bladder Infection, Cystitis)

Physical description: An infection of the urinary tract or bladder caused by an overgrowth of bacteria, fungi, parasites, or viruses. It tends to be more common in women and causes a frequent, urgent desire to urinate, as well as burning pain with urination, blood in the urine, and pain with sexual intercourse.

Energy center(s): Sacral

Nourishment: *Diet*—(1) Drink adequate fluids throughout the day (about eight 8-ounce glasses) and include unsweetened cranberry juice (which prevents the adherence of bacteria to the mucosal lining of the urethra and bladder); (2) Avoid simple sugars. *Supplements*—(1) A multivitamin that contains vitamins A and C and zinc for immune system support; (2) Botanicals such as uva ursi and goldenseal; (3) Probiotics to establish healthy flora; (4) Bioflavonoids for promoting healthy collagen and inflammation.

Emotion(s): Anger, irritation, repression, feeling invaded (all especially with respect to a lover)

Limiting belief(s): It pains me to let go. Flowing is irritating.

Power animal: Fish

Flower essence(s): Walnut

Affirmation(s): I flow. I am open to feelings moving through me. I express myself completely with others.

Visualization: Put your focus on your low back by rubbing your hands together and placing them in that area. Breathe deep and pull your inhale into your low back and hold the breath within your kidneys. Imagine the breath swirls and permeates all the structures responsible for urine production and excretion: your kidneys, ureters, bladder, and urethra. The presence of the breath creates relaxation within these organs.

Now envision that sitting before you is a twenty-ounce bottle of fluid. The fluid is translucent with a reddish tinge, and it radiates a soft, pulsating glow of light. You feel inclined to drink the substance, as you feel that it will help to clear your body of infection, particularly in your urinary tract. So you pick up the flask of fluid and start to drink it slowly, until you have finished the contents.

With your inner vision, see the liquid permeating your inner body, weaving its way into the fluid the cells are bathed in, gathering up any debris within its silky matrix. As it does this, the liquid compartment of your body, which happens to be a majority of your constitution, becomes clear, clean, and revitalized.

Let the liquid find its way to your kidneys. Within your kidneys, the liquid spins its way through the intricate web of small tubes inside, purifying them from any invading bacteria, fungi, or viruses. Any accumulation or debris in the tubules is shed and dumped into the reddish, healing fluid and then moves down into the tubes that exit the kidneys, traveling the path that would normally be traveled by the urine. The glow of the red-colored liquid fills the tubes connecting the kidneys to the bladder and, similar to an outdoor bug light, zaps any microorganisms that occupy this space. The liquid itself creates a soft, protective coating on the inner core of the tube to prevent the adhesion of any new invaders.

Eventually, the liquid light moves through to the bladder, swirling inside like a small whirlpool. The bladder expels any residual, clinging feelings of irritation, holding back, or resentment into the whirl of energy in its space. The environment within the bladder becomes brighter and lighter, less cluttered and dark. Like the tubes that connect to the bladder, it is coated with a sheen layer that imparts courage and wisdom.

With an inhale and a resounding, long exhale, see the reddish liquid exiting your body. The pH of your body has come back into balance, and your internal microflora has been restored to one of health and healing.

Meditation: Meditate in the presence of running water, such as a stream, river, or even a fountain (small or large).

Urticaria (See Hives)

Uterine Fibroids

Physical description: Noncancerous growths that attach in or to the wall of the uterus and that may be stimulated to grow in the presence of excessive estrogen. They vary in size (becoming as large as a grapefruit) and occur in a majority of women throughout their lifetime.

Energy center(s): Sacral

Nourishment: *Diet*—(1) Avoid red meat (beef, pork), dairy products, sugar, alcohol, and caffeine, as these foods may influence liver function. Healthy liver function is needed for ensuring that estrogen levels remain balanced; (2) Include foods high in plant estrogens, such as flaxseed, rye, millet, buckwheat, barley, to name a few. Plant estrogens tend to be weaker than the estrogen in the body, but compete with the body's estrogen and may help reduce some of its detrimental effects; (3) Eat iron-rich vegetable foods, such as kale, spinach and black beans, to replenish iron stores lost in excessive uterine bleeding. *Supplements*—(1) Pancreatic enzymes between meals to assist with breaking down fibrous tissue; (2) Iron supplement, if anemia is present; (3) Essential fatty acids from fish or flaxseed oil to help reduce inflammation and promote immune health; (4) Milk-thistle extract to promote healthy liver function to detoxify excessive estrogen; (5) Supplemental fiber powders to assist in the removal of excessive estrogen via the gut.

Emotion(s): Hurt, sadness, emotional attachment to others

Limiting belief(s): I hold my pain within. I find it difficult to detach from relationships. I am not creative. I put others before myself. It is easier for me to withdraw from others than to deal with the emotions created from my relationship with them.

Power animal: Spider

Flower essence(s): Red Chestnut

Affirmation(s): I embrace my feminine wisdom. I grow into feminine expression. I welcome right relationship. I am creative. I express my hurts.

Visualization: Envision that you dive your hands into your low abdomen to retrieve your uterus. Carefully remove it and put it on a throwing wheel that would be used for crafting pottery. See the shape of your uterus transformed into a bowl-like shape made of red, earthen clay. With your hands and your eyes closed, begin to feel the inner walls of the uterus. Feel it meticulously, inch by inch, to see what form it has taken within you. You may feel some lumps, or fibroids, built into the muscle wall. Notice the texture of the walls; are they thin or thick or somewhere in between?

Your uterus is a creative organ, the wellspring of feminine artistry. Now it is your turn to create with your uterus, using your hands as though you were making your finest pottery. She is ready to be sculpted and perfected to your liking. When you start the spinning wheel moving in slow speed, the sound of a plucked harp fills your ears. Your hands are on either side of the "clay," and you enjoy feeling the texture of your beautiful uterus. You begin running your hands along the sides, smoothing out any imperfections—knots of tissue, adhesions, unevenly textured walls. You do this carefully, purely with your own intuitive, creative sense. You do not even have to use your eyes—just your sense of touch.

Your uterus enjoys being handled in an artistic way. She begins to release any stored tension, unresolved issues, and clustered, unexpressed creativity through your fingertips. You help her tissue to be even and soft. When you feel that you have shaped her to your liking and hers, hold her within your hands and tell her what a beautiful, creative, wholly feminine source she has been in your life. Envision a swirl of sunset-colored energy bathing the inner part of the uterus and the outer, until she is coated in creativity and love.

When you have infused her with what feels important, cup her in your hands and position her back in your low belly in an upright position—not tilted backwards or forwards, but just right, like a teacup poised in its saucer. Place your left hand on this part of your abdomen and invite your natural healer energy to be present here whenever your uterus needs help.

Meditation: Meditate in a seated posture, with your hands cupped deep on your low belly, at the level of the uterus. Focus on the release of blocks or stagnation in your uterus, using your breath as an image to stimulate the flow of the release.

Varicose Veins

Physical description: The formation of swollen, enlarged, twisted veins—typically the superficial veins of the leg. The veins collect pools of blood as a result of their valves becoming damaged and stretched. Aside from being cosmetically disfiguring, varicose veins can cause discomfort, such as a heavy, tired, tight feeling, and can even be painful.

Energy center(s): Root, heart

Nourishment: *Diet*—(1) Focus on high-fiber foods like vegetables (e.g., brussels sprouts, broccoli, peas, sweet potatoes) and fruits (e.g., blackberries, apples, kiwis, prunes) to promote bowel-movement regularity; (2) Eat berries (blackberries, marionberries, blueberries, strawberries, raspberries), because they supply plant compounds that support vein health and structure. *Supplements*—(1) Vitamin C for healthy protein (collagen) that composes veins; (2) Bioflavonoids (take together with vitamin C) to promote healthy vein structure; (3) Supplemental fiber powders, such as psyllium, help keep stools soft and regular; (4) Botanical supplements such as horse chestnut, bilberry, grape seed, and pine bark extract have been used for varicose veins.

Emotion(s): Disappointment

Limiting belief(s): I am collapsing under the weight of my life. I am stuck and unable to move forward. I need to apply pressure to get results. Life is heavy.

Power animal: Antelope

Flower essence(s): Blackberry

Affirmation(s): My energy circulates freely and quickly. I am free and mobile. My life unfolds effortlessly.

Visualization: Close your eyelids, breathe in, and open your inner eyes to a completely different image of yourself. See a large white daisy in the middle of your chest, at the place of your heart. Notice the white, fragile petals responding to the movement of the breath—rhythmically, in and out, in and out. With each inhale you feel more relaxed and at peace, and with every exhale, you are filled with joy and love.

Place your awareness on the underside of the daisy, at the level of the yellow core, at the place where the blossom joins to its stem. Notice the stem of the daisy extending down your torso, and at the base of the torso, you see all of its roots extending out. However, these roots are different than you might find on a typical flower. These roots span an entire network throughout your entire body, forming the circulatory system. Let your inner vision walk through the landscape of this intricate root network. See large roots plunging through your legs and into the earth; see medium-sized roots extending out into the upper and middle body, down the arms, into the neck. From these medium and large roots branch off tinier roots, and even these tiny roots split into several other roots. See your body as a huge flower with a network of roots evenly and strategically placed throughout the body.

Your breath becomes the sunlight that feeds you from within. Your roots circulate nutrients and oxygen to every cell of your body, and take waste products away from the cells, so you feel alive and healthy. Envision the long roots in your legs and see the flow of substances coursing through them, depositing any waste into the earth and distributing any nutrients to your cells, so the cells can be invigorated.

Your heart thrives on the flow of these substances; however, sometimes the roots can become blocked or congested. Scan your root network, especially in your legs, to see whether you have any stagnation or pooling of substances. If you do, imagine your breath coming into your flower. The breath turns into white light and travels throughout the system of roots, creating flow and fluidity and breaking up any blocks. Take your time moving the white light through your entire root system. No block is too big for the white light to penetrate and move. Let the white light move through any pain that may have manifested from any blocks in your roots. Move the pain on through to the earth to transform it into nourishment for the planet.

In your own time, when you are ready, transition from the vision of the roots into a vision of your circulatory system; see them as one and the same. By clearing your roots, you have cleared your blood vessels, including arteries, veins, and capillaries, of any stagnation.

Once you have successfully removed all blocks, allowing all nutrients, oxygen, and waste products to travel through your roots with ease, you will feel an enormous rush of energy and invigoration. With your breath, dive into this tremendous wellspring of energy. Each breath you take allows you to bathe in the endless spring of energy. You drink in its essence until it has pervaded not only your physical body, but also your emotional body, your mental body, and your spiritual body. Give yourself thanks for the gift of movement within that enables you to be healthy. And when you are ready, with calm breath, open your eyes.

Meditation: Practice a mindfulness meditation using a blackberry or blueberry. Set the berry on your tongue and meditate on its healing properties moving through you and strengthening your veins.

Venereal Disease (Sexually Transmitted Disease)

Physical description: A highly contagious disease that results from the transmission of an infectious microorganism (bacteria, fungi, parasite, virus) through sexual contact, usually via semen, vaginal secretions, and/or blood. The infection may be dormant (asymptomatic, or showing no symptoms) or result in bodily changes, such as a herpes blister, vaginal discharge, or genital warts. Common venereal diseases include AIDS (acquired immune deficiency syndrome), chlamydia, genital warts, gonorrhea, genital herpes, and syphilis.

Energy center(s): Root, sacral

Nourishment: *Diet*—(1) Consume nutrient-dense foods that support the immune system, such as legumes, whole grains, and vegetables; (2) Reduce foods that are high in sugars (including alcohol), as they may depress immune system function; (3) Make sure to consume high-quality fats that support the immune system, like omega-3 fats from fish (e.g., salmon), flaxseed oil, nuts (e.g., walnuts), and seeds (e.g., hemp); (4) Eat adequate amounts of protein; (5) For herpes simplex, reduce foods high in arginine, such as chocolate, nuts, and some legumes (e.g., peanut), and include foods high in lysine, such as most vegetables and lean animal-protein sources (e.g., turkey, chicken). *Supplements*—(1) Multivitamin containing vitamin A (anti-infection vitamin), vitamin C, B complex, and zinc; (2) Probiotic supplement for keeping mucosal membranes healthy and balanced in their bacterial populations; (3) Lysine supplementation for those with herpes simplex.

Emotion(s): Shame, guilt

Limiting belief(s): I am not worthy. I am ashamed of my sexuality. I feel guilty for having sexual intercourse. I fear intimacy. I feel vulnerable and full of fear when I open myself to others.

Power animal: Tiger

Flower essence(s): Basil, Hibiscus, Sticky Monkeyflower

Affirmation(s): I am a beautiful, creative being. I embrace my sexuality. I am open to healthy intimacy.

Visualization: Imagine drawing a bath. As warm water fills the bathtub, you add in salts and aromatherapy oils to make the bath even more therapeutic. You undress and step into the warm water, and at once, you start to feel a wave of relaxation move through your body. You carefully sit in the tub, letting your head rest against the back. Warmth permeates your entire being from the outside inwards, and you feel even more relaxed, to the extent that you are able to unwind and dive deeper into your subconscious mind.

Let down your guard to explore some aspects of your boundaries within relationships—information residing in the territory of the root and sacral chakras. Fix your attention on the lower part of your torso, under your navel. With your subconscious as a vehicle, see if you can see any ribbons of energy extending outward towards people that you have had some degree of intimacy with, including sexual encounters. If those relationships have ended, roll up those ribbons of energy into your lower torso, keeping them tucked tight within you. Do this sequentially for every relationship you have had that has completed itself in the physical world but is not necessarily finished from an emotional perspective. Rather than have your energy moving outward for a nonexistent relationship, direct it back inward to increase emotional reserves in your low belly.

Once you feel that you've completed this activity, move your awareness into the root-sacral chakra terrain. Gather up all the energy you've collected and transform it into a flower garden in this space. Envision this garden as being lush and abundant with roses, daisies, lilacs, lilies, and any other flowers that you choose. All the flowers thrive and live harmoniously within the garden. The sun beams down on the flowers, and you absorb in this radiant, photonic energy, which casts light on anything that has remained hidden, dormant, or in a shadow. Invite your ability to be creative, playful, and sexual to emerge from your root-sacral chakra. Let it be bathed in the healing light of the sun, which clears any outdated, unserving patterns and allows your ability to dance back into balance.

Once you feel that this part of you moves to the rhythm of who you are, zoom in on the activity of your immune system and your body's boundaries, making sure that they kept strong. Examine the boundary around your body and ensure that there is a tight net of safety and exchange around you. Let go of anything caught within this net that serves you incorrectly. Infuse the intensity of the sunlight in your root-sacral chakra garden into the whole of your being, radiating it through to bring in the element of strength and wholeness to your immune system. Feel your entire immune army being fortified by the sun. Breathe in this reserve of energy, and as you do, feel the energy of the cleansing power of the bath salts penetrate your being to help your body defend itself from any bacteria, viruses, microbes, or fungi. With the next breath, see your body's boundary being infused with the energy of the essential oils that you used in your bath. The aroma and oil keep your body protected and clear of interference.

When you feel ready, step out of the bath, letting the bathwater, and anything that released from you into the water, make their way down the drain. Dry yourself off with a towel of forgiveness and truth. And feel alive, strong, and well in your new skin!

Meditation: If you are in a relationship with another person, engage in a short meditation together. Facing each other while seated cross-legged, meditate on the balance of energy that you exchange between yourselves.

If you are not in a relationship, meditate on balancing your feminine and masculine sides. Focus on the left (the feminine) side of your body first and your right (the masculine) side second. Bring the two aspects of your nature together by meditating on their unification.

Viral Infection

Physical description: A virus is a small organism (smaller than a fungus or bacterium) that requires a host (e.g., person, animal, or plant) to live. It can invade the human body through ingestion, inhalation, insect bites, or sexual contact. Invasion by a virus can be short lived, as with a common cold or influenza, or long lived and latent, like herpes viruses are. The presence of a virus in the human body taxes the immune system.

Energy center(s): Root

Nourishment: *Diet*—(1) Reduce or eliminate consumption of all types of sugars, as sugar intake may depress the activity of the immune system; (2) Investigate the presence of food allergies with your healthcare practitioner. *Supplements*—General multivitamin containing vitamin A, vitamin C, and zinc.

Emotion(s): Insecurity, hurt, regret

Limiting belief(s): I am exposed. I am vulnerable. Others attack me, and I cannot defend myself. I am overwhelmed.

Power animal: Bear

Flower essence(s): Garlic

Affirmation(s): I am strong and invincible. I am invigorated with life force. Everything occurs with perfection.

Visualization: Concentrate on grounding firmly into the earth through your feet. Move your feet back and forth slightly until you have found a comfortable position. With your attention at your feet, invoke healing energy, in the form of liquid light, to stream up from the crystalline core at the heart of the earth. Move it quickly through the layers of the earth's crust to arrive at the soles of your feet. Draw it up into your bones and let it penetrate the bone marrow. See the liquid light traveling up your legs and pooling in your pelvic basin. Have tiny rivulets flow through the body, weaving their way among cells so every cell is touched by their presence.

This liquid light is so luminescent and bright that it is able to zap anything that is detrimental to you, including, and especially, viruses. Observe how it begins to destroy any and all viruses inhabiting your being that are not of the highest good. Give it the time it needs to locate all the viruses.

Once these viruses are killed, they are transported into the pool of light in your pelvic basin. Their energy is transmuted into that of protection, boundaries, and vigilance. The pooled, transformed light begins to spin around clockwise in your pelvic region and then streaks of it are sent, like shooting stars, up into your torso, into your head, into your arms, and into your legs. Every part of you is saturated with protection from any unnecessary invaders. Your immune system is strengthened by the presence of the healing white light. It becomes charged and active, ready to defend your body systems appropriately.

These shafts of light, radiating out in five directions—through your head, two arms, and two legs—now go beyond the boundaries of your physical body. The light pours out from these five directions, creating radiance; a glow of this protective light spreads all around you in the form of an egg shape. The material is like fine mist and will allow that which is good, true, and beautiful to enter your sphere. It will ward off anything that will drain you of your vital energy. If you need to renew and reset your protective sphere at any time in the future, rapidly raise your hands simultaneously, clap them over your head, and let them fall quickly at your sides. Repeat this action at least ten to fifteen times to renew your sphere and stimulate your lymph.

Meditation: Envision a glowing, white, protective mist and meditate within it for one to two minutes, four times daily (every three to four hours).

Vision Loss

Physical description: A complete or partial loss of sight, which may be due to diseases of the retina (e.g., macular degeneration), optic nerve (e.g., glaucoma), or changes caused in other anatomical structures of the eye, like the lens (e.g., cataract).

Energy center(s): Third eye

Nourishment: *Diet*—(1) Eat green and yellow fruits and vegetables, like broccoli, spinach, and leafy greens; (2) Emphasize low-glycemic-index foods, such as legumes, whole grains, and lean meats. (Salmon is an excellent choice for the eyes because of its omega-3 content.); (3) Avoid overcooking foods. *Supplements*—(1) Lutein; (2) Antioxidant vitamins like vitamins C and E; (3) Zinc; (4) Fish or flaxseed oil.

Emotion(s): Denial, dread of what is to come

Limiting belief(s): I am blinded to my intuition. I turn my eyes away from my internal wisdom. My life is darkened and obscure.

Power animal: Eagle

Flower essence(s): Queen Anne's Lace

Affirmation(s): I see clearly. I am open to the possibility of my inner vision. The light of my intuition shines forth. I receive insight from higher dimensions that enables me to have perspective. My life is full of clarity. I am in-sight-full.

Visualization: Close your eyes and tilt your gaze towards your third eye—slightly up towards the middle of your forehead, right above your eyebrows. With this eye, you have expansive vision, spanning throughout many dimensions and galaxies. It enables you to see the minute detail in very large objects that are far away. Your third eye is all knowing, all seeing, and endows you with the special ability to see even past physical structures into their origin.

With this space, envision a spiraling microgalaxy of violet stars that produce an incredibly bright violet light. This light is the spirit of your internal vision, and it guides you to your higher path.

Allow this light to shine directly down into your right eye. The light caresses all the structures of your eye, working from the outside to the inside. It clears away all clouded vision, any damage to the eye, and restores the eye so it functions perfectly. The light also coats the optic nerve in the back of the eye, enabling its wiring to the brain to be seamless. The right eye basks in the glow of this sparkling light, absorbing its healing rays.

Once this eye has become saturated with the light and is healed to the extent that it is able, the light then travels horizontally over to the left eye, coating that eye with its luminescence, brightening it from the outer layer and slowly penetrating through to the inner core of the eye. Like the right eye, the left eye has been cleared of anything that prevented it from seeing near and far. The optic nerve is bathed in the glittering violet light, and it is restored to health.

The violet light now unifies both eyes, allowing them to function together perfectly. The bright light travels back up to the third eye, forming a pyramid of purple light between the three eyes. The purple light pulses and circulates from the third eye to the other eyes, nourishing them with insight, imagination, intuition, and clear vision of objects and events near and far. The light concentrates back into the third-eye center, and slowly and gently, its glow recedes. You open your eyes, welcoming your new vision!

Meditation: Go within silently and meditate on your third eye, especially at the end of the day before bedtime. With your fingertips, gently tap the area around the eyes.

Worry

Physical description: A state in which a person is mentally preoccupied with distressing thoughts or concern. Often, this state is associated with an event yet to happen or the effects of an event that has already occurred. Worry for brief periods of time may be beneficial for motivating someone to a healthy action, but when it is extended, it can turn into anxiety and nervousness.

Energy center(s): Root, solar plexus, third eye

Nourishment: *Diet*—Limit or eliminate alcohol, caffeine, and sugar-containing foods. *Supplements*—(1) Balanced mineral supplement, preferably one that contains adequate magnesium (aim for 200 to 400 mg per day); (2) B-complex vitamin for ensuring adequate synthesis of neurotransmitters and balanced metabolism; (3) Several calming botanicals, such as hops, valerian, passionflower, and chamomile, are also available.

Emotion(s): Worry, fear, dread

Limiting belief(s): I feel helpless. I am inadequate. I am unable to defend myself against the unknown. I am all alone.

Flower essence(s): Filaree, Gorse

Affirmation(s): I am perfectly equipped to handle any situation presented to me. I trust my abilities. I believe in myself.

Visualization: Lie down in a comfortable place, with your arms at your sides, your legs stretched long, and your chest open. Imagine yourself floating, face up, in a body of water. Take a deep breath, and as you do, see a lifesaver, a buoyant tube, in front of you. As you take hold of it, it floats you into another realm of consciousness and relaxation. With each breath, you are reeled in closer and closer to a shore, until you feel grounded and centered.

Now shift your awareness to the full expanse of your body. You are going to move through a series of exercises that will help you to let go of everything that weighs you down and burdens you. The first step in that direction is to do a whole-body purge and release. So with your whole body spread out very relaxed, take a breath in, and as you do, tighten everything as best you can. Squint your eyes, scrunch your face, tighten your shoulders, flex your chest muscles and arms, and make fists with both hands. Tighten your abdomen, pulling it in towards your middle; tighten your legs and knees, and flex your feet. Be in a place of pure, constricted energy, and as you are, gather up all the strands, flecks, blobs, and balls of worry from all these tightened areas. Let them be squeezed out of your tissues, organs, and cells.

And after just a couple of seconds of holding the tight feeling, let go completely, starting with the top of your body and relaxing your face, neck, shoulders, arms. Open your hands, and let your belly go. Relax your legs and knees, and unflex your feet. You may feel this release as an ocean wave washing over you—only instead of a wave of water, a wave of relaxation trickles through your being.

And with this wave, all worries, preoccupations, expectations, and fear rise from you, like a multitude of kites waving in the blue sky. See them soaring upwards. And with a deep inhale, see yourself letting go of all the threads. Surrender all of these to the sky. Watch them become smaller and smaller, more and more distant, until they finally disappear.

Observe the difference you feel in your body. Perform this activity as many times as you need to feel completely and utterly relaxed and relieved of worry.

Since much of our worry is created through our thought patterns, let's now travel into the matrix of the mind for a moment. Imagine the mind is an attic of a beautiful house. But this attic has become dusty, cluttered, and dark. Breathe into this space, and as you do so, see all the dust whirl together into a pile in the center of the room. Open all the windows in this space to air it out and bring in sunshine and warmth. Remove all the clutter by shuffling it into place in an organized way. All books go back on shelves, arranged alphabetically so you can find them easily again. Other boxes or objects are stacked neatly, and you dispose of anything not in alignment with who you are. Saturate this space with healing light and positivity, pushing out all fears and worry patterns that you may have been programmed with. Start from scratch and fill your mind only with patterns that are good, true, and beautiful.

At this point, feel the flow of being in the present moment. You have shed all remnants from the past that are connected to worry and all threads from the future that weave a blanket of worry. You are free of fear and distress. Feel the freedom of the potential of the present moment filling your being.

Meditation: (1) Participating in a regularly scheduled group meditation is helpful, as it gives you a network of community support, which is important in reducing worry.

(2) Meditate on the support network in your life through silent reflection or by writing cards to those who have been present in your life and made a difference.

Yeast Infection (Candida Albicans Overgrowth)

Physical description: An overgrowth of the fungus *Candida albicans* in the body, particularly in moist, mucosal tissues, such as in the intestine, nasal passages, and vagina. The overgrowth is typically due to impaired immune function and is promoted by a prolonged use of antibiotics, consumption of a high-sugar diet, lack of activity, stress, and poor sleep. It can result in a variety of symptoms, including changes in bowel patterns, itching, joint pain, mucous congestion, and rashes.

Energy center(s): Root, sacral

Nourishment: *Diet*—(1) Eliminate refined or simple sugars (such as fruit juice, or products that contain any number of sugars, including sucrose, honey, corn syrup, dextrose, and maple syrup, to name a few) and starchy foods (pastas, bread); (2) Eliminate foods that contain mold and yeast, such as alcohol (all types), cheeses (all), and dried fruits and nuts; (3) Aim to eat vegetables, lean protein sources, and sparing amounts of fruit (better fruits include berries of all types, apples, and pears, if they are in season). *Supplements*—(1) Probiotics to help balance the gut flora; (2) Natural antifungals, such as goldenseal, Oregon grape, barberry, and garlic. *Note that several antifungals should not be used in pregnancy; check with your healthcare professional;* (3) Fibers such as psyllium help eliminate gut toxins.

Emotion(s): Apathy, anxiety, feeling overwhelmed

Limiting belief(s): I am depleted. My life feels out of control. People take my energy from me. My boundaries are weak. My life has been overtaken by a lack of joy.

Power animal: Frog

Flower essence(s): Pink Yarrow, Red Chestnut, Yarrow

Affirmation(s): I am clear, free, and clean of that which serves me incorrectly. I live in joy. I take in that which nourishes me. I have healthy boundaries.

Visualization: When you breathe in, imagine your breath as a population of tiny pink bubbles. And as you inhale, see these bubbles coming first into your chest and then into your lower gut, filling your entire torso with a sense of lightness.

Now transition your attention to two dazzling, yellow-colored receptacles situated at the bottom of each foot. Their purpose is to take away all that serves you incorrectly. There is enough room in those containers for all you need to release. They shine two strong rays of light very brightly throughout your body, illuminating and dispelling all fear and worry from your being. You feel a sense of peace knowing that they are available to you, and you realize that you can call upon them to assist in removing whatever is needed at any time.

You notice a horizontal, white laser light, about six feet in length and about three inches in diameter, positioned at the top of your head. This light will clear you of any yeast by infusing your body with a potent vibration that casts out all yeast organisms, causing them to fall into the golden receptacles at the bottom of your feet. As you slowly inhale, the light moves over the region of your head, filling it with iridescent, glowing white, healing light that immediately destroys any fungal, bacterial, or viral organisms that are not helpful to your body or soul. In an instant, all of these organisms fall at lightning speed through your body to the receptacles below your feet. At once, your mind feels clearer; you notice you can breathe fully, and your hearing is acute and clear.

With your next breath, the laser light moves through the throat, through the upper shoulders, and down your arms and into your fingertips. You notice all the organisms held within you for so long are now being electrified and sent quickly through your fingertips into the two containers. You begin to feel a surge of energy running through you. Your neck and shoulders feel more fluid, and the joints in your hands move with ease.

The glowing, blinding white light moves into your torso and, starting at the upper body, releases pathogenic organisms from your lungs, blood vessels, and heart tissue. It then travels into the digestive organs, clearing away all dampness and darkness and organisms that have made these areas their home, but that serve you incorrectly. Ribbons of the white light travel through the extent of your digestive tract, enabling the gut tissue to heal. The light eradicates all unhealthy bugs by sending them straight into the brilliant yellow containers of transformation. At once, your gut feels free and light, relieved of any heaviness, bloating, or congestion.

The next inhale brings this light spiraling through your reproductive organs, clearing this area of any unwanted organisms. Immediately they fall away down through the legs and out through the feet, into the receptacles. The receptacles glow as they receive all these organisms. The light travels sequentially down the legs, over and through the knees, and out the feet. Every single unwanted, unhealthy fungus, bacteria, and virus has been cleared from your system completely.

All that no longer serves your being sits in the glowing yellow receptacles, and in a moment, they transform into two bright orbs of yellow light. Both have the intensity of the light of the sun, and they burn away all the stuck, unserving, stagnant organisms from your body until they exist no more. You are free and filled with white, pure light that causes your body to vibrate at a high frequency. It is so bright that the light filters through every pore of your body, creating a layer around your body that is sacred and impenetrable.

Take a deep breath in, giving gratitude to the healing of your body that has just occurred. With your exhale, hear the sound of a magnificent, resonant gong. The rich sound of the gong shimmers and radiates throughout every cell of your body, sounding a call specific for your immune system. At the next gong sound, the entire army of your immune system lines up and becomes strengthened. And, with a deep breath, you disperse the immune system's soldiers, the white blood cells, to the places of the body where they are most needed. You feel secure having them available to you. They are functioning better than they have in years.

You feel a new energy pulsing within you—that of your eternal self, free of any debris and stagnation. Allow this part of you to enter into your everyday awareness.

Meditation: While sitting in stillness, imagine what your personal boundary looks like around you. Is it present? Is it open or torn in some places? Or is it too solid and impenetrable? Form your personal boundary in your mind's eye, and once it has been set, meditate on it for a couple of minutes in the morning and in the evening to strengthen it.

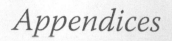

Appendices

Emotional Continuums

If you are feeling *sad,* ask yourself whether you can define your sadness as any of the following:	Do you feel guilty? Do you feel ashamed? Do you feel depressed? Do you feel lonely? Do you feel bored? Do you feel tired? Do you feel full of regret? Do you feel apathetic? Do you feel isolated?
If you are feeling *mad,* ask yourself whether you can define your anger as any of the following:	Do you feel hurt? Do you feel rage? Do you feel hateful? Do you feel critical? Do you feel distant and cold? Do you feel cynical? Do you feel frustrated? Do you feel jealous? Do you feel competitive? Do you feel irritated? Do you feel suspicious and untrusting? Do you feel overwhelmed?

If you are feeling *fearful*, ask yourself whether you can define your fear as any of the following:

Do you feel confused?
Do you feel helpless?
Do you feel rejected?
Do you feel insecure?
Do you feel anxious?
Do you feel discouraged?
Do you feel inadequate?
Do you feel embarrassed?
Do you feel pessimistic?

If you are feeling *happy*, ask yourself whether you can define your happiness as any of the following:

Do you feel excited?
Do you feel energetic?
Do you feel cheerful?
Do you feel creative?
Do you feel abundant?
Do you feel joyful?
Do you feel playful?
Do you feel content?
Do you feel thankful?

Power Animals and Their Significance

Animal	Characteristics, qualities, symbolism
Ant	Hard-working, social, working for a cause, letting go of outcome
Antelope	Agile, adaptable, quick moving, grace
Bear	Healing, strength, flexibility, protection, harnessing messages from dreams
Beaver	Harmonious, problem-solver, fertile, home-builder
Bee	Determination, community, momentum, guardian
Buffalo	Wise, ancestral knowledge, protection, sacredness, grounded
Bull	Assurance, potent, present, earth-loving
Butterfly	Transformation, beauty, illumination, uniqueness, carefree

Cat	Agility, curiosity, clever, mysterious, playful
Cow	Gentle, compassion, serene, peaceful, fair
Coyote	Teaching, humor, the unexpected, laughter, duality
Crocodile	Birth, fertility, exploration, subtle, primal feminine power
Crow	Wayshower, magic, abundance, links physical and spiritual realities
Deer	Gentleness, humility, love, forgiveness
Dog	Loyalty, devotion, service
Dolphin	Ancient wisdom, grace, divine guidance, evolution, enlightened expression
Dove	Peaceful, inspiration, purity, clarity, illumination
Dragonfly	Inner vision, gathering perspectives, transformation, swift
Eagle	Creation, source, journey into the unknown, surrender, truth
Elephant	Wisdom, knowledge, insight, venerable, service, majestic
Elk	Transforms weaknesses into strengths, endurance, warrior energy
Fish	Fluidity, peaceful, surrender, guidance
Fox	Strategic, clever, wisdom, nobility

Frog	Cleansing, purity, observation, quick, regeneration
Goat	Feeling secure, ambition, curiosity, endurance, accomplishment
Hawk	Protective, mother-energy, visionary, observer
Heron	Femininity, regeneration, depth, delicate
Horse	Freedom, adventure, strength, brave
Hummingbird	Happiness, freedom, sweetness
Lamb	Gentle, kind, non-judgmental
Leopard	Investigative, stealth, mystery
Lion	Courage, heart-centered, radiance, regal
Lizard	Experience, satisfaction, ancient wisdom
Monkey	Playfulness, humor, courage
Moose	Determined, knowing one's values, focused
Mouse	Order, organizing details, preparing, quietude
Otter	Unique, eccentric, looking at blind spots, insightful
Owl	Wisdom, observing, cautious, feminine
Panther	Ferocity, understanding the shadow side, confidence, agility
Peacock	Wisdom, intuition, beauty, expression

Pig	Loyalty, honesty, forgiveness
Polar bear	Peaceful, self-acceptance, powerful
Porcupine	Stand one's ground, confidence, turning adversity into opportunity
Rabbit	Warmth, fertility, rebirth, change
Raccoon	Embracing our shadow, resourceful, tenacious
Ram	Rebirth, renewal, new beginnings
Raven	Shape-shifter, messenger of the spirit world, independent, instinctual
Salmon	Instinct, internal quest, overcoming challenges
Sheep	Caring, sharing, connected to others
Skunk	Protective, peaceful, discriminating
Snake	Liberation, rebirth, agelessness, mystical wisdom, ancient
Spider	Feminine energy, protector, guide, patterns possibilities
Squirrel	Abundance, trust, prepared
Swan	Acceptance, willingness, adept, graceful, exquisiteness
Tiger	Creative power, sexuality, strength
Turkey	Gratitude, objectivity, generosity

Turtle	Caution, perseverance, security, protection
Whale	Integrity, synthesis, depth of knowledge
Wolf	Movement, evaluation, bountiful inner reserve, vigilance

Flower Essences and Their Qualities

Flower Essence	Characteristics, qualities, symbolism
Agrimony *Agrimonia eupatoria*	Allows the true self to surface, authenticity
Aloe Vera *Aloe vera*	Helps to cool down a strong internal drive and fiery ambition
Alpine Lily *Lilium parvum*	Assists in the integration of the feminine aspect with the whole being
Angel's Trumpet *Datura candida*	Helps in surrendering and letting go
Angelica *Angelica archangelica*	Connects body to spirit; creates a better balance between the physical and spiritual aspects of one's being
Arnica *Arnica mollis*	Helps in the recovery from trauma or injury

Aspen *Populus tremula*	Transforms anxiety from oversensitivity into assurance
Baby Blue Eyes *Nemophila menziesii*	Transforms an approach to life that is too independent, with fear around survival and trust, into one that is interdependent and trusting
Basil *Ocimum basilicum*	Aligns sexuality and spirituality issues in one's being
Beech *Fagus sylvatica*	Relaxes perfectionistic tendencies
Black Cohosh *Cimicifuga racemosa*	Brings an element of peace into a turbulent life
Black-eyed Susan *Rudbeckia hirta*	Allows the ability to look at buried wounds or shadows in one's life
Blackberry *Rubus ursinus*	Moves one from stagnation into action
Bleeding Heart *Dicentra formosa*	Helps mend a grief-stricken heart
Borage *Borago officinalis*	Creates light-heartedness
Buttercup *Ranunculus occidentalis*	Elevates self-worth
Calendula *Calendula officinalis*	Heightens a feeling of genuine warmth towards others
California Pitcher Plant *Darlingtonia californica*	Helps develop instinct

California Poppy *Eschscholzia californica*	Grounds one in the realities of life and encourages inner confidence
California Wild Rose *Rosa californica*	Encourages risk taking and enthusiasm towards life
Calla Lily *Zantedeschia aethiopica*	Allows for a sense of sexual identity
Canyon Dudleya *Dudleya cymosa*	Releases one from heightened drama and into practical, realistic living
Cayenne *Capsicum annuum*	Imparts motivation and renewed interest
Centaury *Centaurium erythraea* *Centaurium umbellatum*	Balances taking care of self with that of others; puts one in touch with one's needs and provides the confidence to implement these needs
Cerato *Ceratostigma* *willmottiana*	Assists in trusting one's decisions and opinions by enhancing connection to one's inner wisdom
Chamomile *Matricaria recutita*	Smoothes the flow of emotions through the physical and subtle bodies
Chaparral *Larrea tridentata*	Helps to uproot troubles or fearful trauma lodged in the subconscious mind
Cherry Plum *Prunus cerasifera*	Unwinds one's being from the tension associated with stress
Chestnut Bud *Aesculus hippocastanum*	Encourages harnessing the wisdom from past life experiences and applying it to future life situations

Chicory *Cichorium intybus*	Releases the need for attention and encourages inner strength and validation
Chrysanthemum *Chrysanthemum morifolium*	Assists in moving one through crisis
Clematis *Clematis vitalba*	Brings one's internal and external lives into balance
Corn *Zea mays*	Comforts and anchors one in their physical surroundings
Cosmos *Cosmos bipinnatus*	Facilitates streamlined communication
Crab Apple *Malus sylvestris*	Releases an obsessive need for perfection and purification
Dandelion *Taraxacum officinale*	Encourages going with the flow of life and releasing any tension due to overwork
Deerbrush *Ceanothus integerrimus*	Helps one to be authentic in his or her actions and words
Dill *Anethum graveolens*	Prevents sensory input from a taxing environment from overwhelming one and assists one in "digesting" events
Dogwood *Cornus nuttallii*	Helps one to move with grace and ease
Easter Lily *Lilium longiflorum*	Releases any inner conflict about one's sexuality
Echinacea *Echinacea purpurea*	Encourages one's inner strength and healing from past trauma

Elm *Ulmus procera*	Lessens the feeling of burden and expectations
Evening Primrose *Oenothera hookeri*	Brings forth a sense of compassion and love for others and self
Fairy Lantern *Calochortus albus*	Encourages the inner child self to be integrated with the adult self
Fawn Lily *Erythronium purpurascens*	Allows one's time spent in spiritual activities to be integrated with physical life
Filaree *Erodium cicutarium*	Moves one away from worrying about details and gives one overall perspective
Forget-me-not *Myosotis sylvatica*	Facilitates a feeling of deep connection with others
Fuchsia *Fuchsia hybrida*	Allows for the unearthing of deep, authentic emotions within oneself
Garlic *Allium sativum*	Invigorates one's defenses and life force
Gentian *Gentiana amarella*	Encourages faith and optimism
Golden Ear Drops *Dicentra chrysanta*	Unravels buried childhood memories and allows for the expression of real feelings
Golden Yarrow *Achillea filipendulina*	Promotes self-confidence, particularly in public settings
Goldenrod *Solidago californica*	Enhances self-acceptance and encourages inner exploration

Gorse *Ulex europaeus*	Establishes trust and faith in difficult situations
Heather *Calluna vulgaris*	Encourages inner security and fulfillment rather than resorting to others for validation
Hibiscus *Hibiscus rosa-sinensis*	Assists in the integration of intimacy with sexual intercourse, helps develop a sense of safety around sexual encounters
Holly *Ilex aquifolium*	Relaxes competitive and jealous feelings and encourages compassion and love towards others
Honeysuckle *Lonicera caprifolium*	Releases attachment to past circumstances that keep one bound from going further
Hornbeam *Carpinus betulus*	Transforms fatigue and boredom into a renewed feeling of perspective on life
Hound's Tongue *Cynoglossum grande*	Enhances intuition and imagination
Impatiens *Impatiens glandulifera*	Brings forth patience and a sense of inner peace that situations unfold as they need to
Indian Paintbrush *Castilleja miniata*	Balances one's sense of creative expression
Indian Pink *Silene californica*	Helps one to regain inner centeredness
Iris *Iris douglasiana* *Iris versicolor*	Gives one a magical, mystical outlook on life rather than one that is dull and mundane

Lady's Slipper *Cypripedium parviflorum* *Cypripedium reginae*	Helps one to live his or her life's passion and to regain personal power
Larch *Larix decidua*	Replaces an overly critical nature with one that is forgiving and confident
Larkspur *Delphinium nuttallianum*	Encourages a healthy sense of authority and leadership
Lavender *Lavendula officinalis*	Relieves one of mental tension and the ability to balance physical excesses and spiritual withdrawal
Lotus *Nelumbo nucifera*	Balances one's spiritual self with the other aspects of the self (physical, emotional, mental)
Love-lies-bleeding *Amaranthus caudatus*	Relieves physical suffering, uncovers the deep meaning of illness, and reveals what one is unwilling to look at
Madia *Madia elegans*	Enhances mental focus and enables a mindset that is able to complete a project
Mallow *Sidalcea glauscens*	Makes it easy to get along with and be open to other people
Manzanita *Arctostaphylos viscida*	Releases one from bodily abuse through addictions; encourages self-love and body-mind-spirit harmony
Mariposa Lily *Calochortus leichtlinii*	Encourages the restoration of an ability to nurture one's self and others; heals wounds connected to one's mother or mothering
Milkweed *Asclepias cordifolia*	Assists one in developing a healthy independent spirit

Mimulus *Mimulus guttatus*	Enables one to savor the joy in life experiences and to release nagging worries
Morning Glory *Ipomoea purpurea*	Restores the natural body rhythm and dissolves interference to feeling one's vitality
Mountain Pennyroyal *Monardella odoratissima*	Removes transference of other people's concerns and perceptions; helps to release that which is "not self"
Mountain Pride *Penstemon newberryi*	Sparks one's personal power; sheds insecurity and shyness
Mugwort *Artemisia douglasiana*	Helps to balance one's intuition and synchronize it with everyday events
Mustard *Sinapsis arvensis*	Transforms a cloud of deep depression into one of greater understanding and light
Nasturtium *Tropaeolum majus*	Balances intellectual processes with compassion, relieves overthinking, encourages becoming more heart centered
Nicotiana *Nicotiana alata*	Releases the need for external stimuli to help relax, encourages one to be his or her true self
Oak *Quercus robur*	Enhances work-life balance, dissipates exhaustion due to overwork
Olive *Olea europaea*	Encourages physical vitality
Oregon grape *Berberis aquifolium*	Brings forth trust

Penstemon *Penstemon davidsonii*	Instills faith, helps one to gain perspective and clarity
Peppermint *Mentha piperita*	Removes the need for external stimuli for energy, revives the self
Pine *Pinus sylvestris*	Helps transform blame and guilt from past events into learning that helps one move forward with ease
Pink Monkeyflower *Mimulus lewisii*	Helps mend one's sense of vulnerability, strengthens the heart
Pink Yarrow *Achillea millefolium* var. *rubra*	Balances emotions within the self, helps establish emotional boundaries with others
Poison Oak *Toxicodendron diversiloba*	Encourages a sense of safety and reduces unnecessary barriers to forming intimate relationships
Pomegranate *Punica granatum*	Helps women to balance work-home dynamics
Pretty Face *Triteleia ixioides*	Enhances acceptance of one's physical body
Purple Monkeyflower *Mimulus kelloggii*	Establishes an authentic path of spirituality for one's self
Quaking Grass *Briza maxima*	Helps one to harmonize with others in a group setting
Queen Anne's Lace *Daucus carota*	Promotes clarity in how one sees other people, enhances eye health
Quince *Chaenomeles speciosa*	Releases the burden of caretaking, encourages nurturing

Rabbitbrush *Chrysothamnus* *nauseosus*	Harmonizes the details of living with the big picture of life, imbues one with a sense of perspective
Red Chestnut *Aesculus carnea*	Releases unhealthy emotional attachment to others, promotes healthy relationship boundaries
Red Clover *Trifolium pratense*	Removes dread and negativity, encourages individual identity
Rock Rose *Helianthemum* *nummularium*	Infuses one with courage and tenacity
Rosemary *Rosmarinus officinalis*	Helps one to feel completely in his or her body and in the present moment
Sage *Salvia officinalis*	Releases one from any regret associated with the history of a life experience, encourages the extraction of wisdom in all events
Sagebrush *Artemisia tridentata*	Encourages release on the physical level
Saguaro *Carnegiea giganteus*	Helps one embrace family tradition and lineage, harmonizes one's individuality within a group
Saint John's Wort *Hypericum perforatum*	Balances light and dark aspects in one's life and brings forth insight
Scarlet Monkeyflower *Mimulus cardinalis*	Encourages clear communication and the transformation of anger
Scleranthus *Scleranthus annuus*	Helps one to anchor into one's full self

Scotch broom *Cytisus scoparius*	Brings forth hope
Self-heal *Prunella vulgaris*	Encourages finding solutions for healing and wellness
Shasta Daisy *Chrysanthemum maximum*	Helps one to make sense of the big picture and to balance one's analytical abilities
Shooting Star *Dodecatheon hendersonii*	Gives one the sense of being at home on earth
Snapdragon *Antirrhinum majus*	Promotes careful speech and communication (right use of voice)
Star of Bethlehem *Ornithogalum umbellatum*	Removes stored stresses and enables the inner light of peace and strength to shine from within
Star Thistle *Centaurea solstitialis*	Promotes generosity of material goods
Star Tulip *Calochortus tolmiei*	Connects one with their inner, intuitive voice
Sticky Monkeyflower *Mimulus aurantiacus*	Balances one's sexuality, opens one up to vulnerability without fear
Sunflower *Helianthus annuus*	Develops one's identity and sense of self, removes conflict and tension with men in one's life
Sweet Chestnut *Castanea sativa*	Diminishes despair and fills one with hope and faith
Sweet Pea *Lathyrus latifolus*	Cultivates physical stability, helps one develop a sense of home

Tansy *Tanacetum vulgare*	Motivates one to achieve their full potential
Tiger Lily *Lilium humboldtii*	Moves one from being separate to feeling connected to others, balances masculine and feminine energy
Trillium *Trillium chloropetalum*	Lessens unhealthy ambition and overwhelming feelings of striving to survive
Trumpet Vine *Campsis tagliabuana*	Harmonizes the voice to express creatively
Vervain *Verbena officinalis*	Reduces an overaggressive nature, opens one to the opinions and beliefs of others
Vine *Vitis vinifera*	Balances willpower and enhances surrender to a higher goal
Violet *Viola odorata*	Instills self-esteem in social settings
Walnut *Juglans regia*	Releases one from stagnation and unhealthy habitual behavior, helps one to flow forward
Water Violet *Hottonia palustris*	Helps one develop humility in working with others and to be respectful of differing opinions and backgrounds
White Chestnut *Aesculus hippocastanum*	Quiets the mind of busy thoughts and agitation, promotes healthy sleep and calmness
Wild Oat *Bromus ramosus*	Enables one to find calling in his or her work
Wild Rose *Rose canina*	Helps one to recover from setbacks

Willow *Salix vitellina*	Releases resentment and grudges, encourages flexibility
Yarrow *Achillea millefolium*	Restores one's boundaries and ability to be in harmony with the environment
Yellow Star Tulip *Calochortus monophyllus*	Helps one to open to his or her empathetic nature
Yerba Santa *Eriodictyon californium*	Opens one to possibilities and to releasing grief or tightness in the chest, enables one to breathe deeply
Zinnia *Zinnia elegans*	Releases the seriousness of life and opens one to their inner child

Source: Modified from *Choosing Flower Essences: An Assessment Guide* by Patricia Kaminski, published by the Flower Essence Society, 1996.

Anatomical Sketch of the Human Body

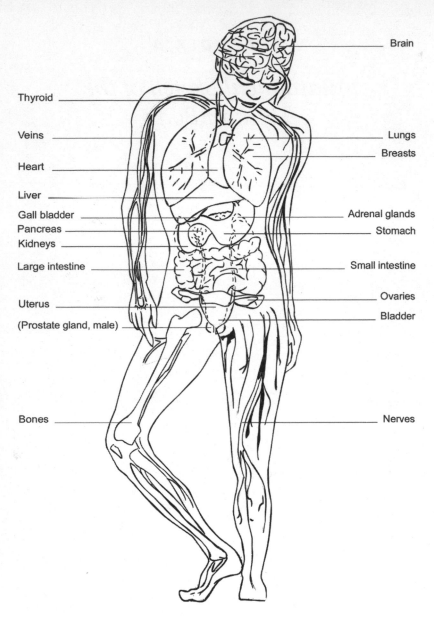

Brain

Thyroid

Veins

Heart

Liver

Gall bladder

Pancreas

Kidneys

Large intestine

Uterus

(Prostate gland, male)

Lungs

Breasts

Adrenal glands

Stomach

Small intestine

Ovaries

Bladder

Bones

Nerves

Main organs of the human body.

APPENDIX E

Positive Emotion Weekly Tracking Checklist

Instructions: At the end of the day, mark with an X any positive emotions that you exhibited.

	SUNDAY	MONDAY	TUESDAY	WEDNESDAY	THURSDAY	FRIDAY	SATURDAY
Able to express self							
Appreciative							
Authentic							
Aware							
Balanced							
Compassionate							
Courageous							
Creative							
Daring							
Energetic							
Exuberant							
Forgiving							
Grateful							
Happy							
Helpful							
Honest							
Interested							
Joyful							
Loving							
Optimistic							
Peaceful							
Playful							
Relaxed							
Self-accepting							
Solutions-oriented							

Bibliography

Chapter 1: What Is Quantum Healing?

Bertisch SM, Wee CC, Phillips RS, McCarthy EP. Alternative mind-body therapies used by adults with medical conditions. *J Psychosom Res.* 2009 Jun;66(6):511–9. Epub 2009 Mar 3.

Carlson LE, Speca M, Faris P, Patel KD. One year pre-post intervention follow-up of psychological, immune, endocrine and blood pressure outcomes of mindfulness-based stress reduction (MBSR) in breast and prostate cancer outpatients. *Brain Behav Immun.* 2007 Nov;21(8):1038–49.

Cohen S, Janicki-Deverts D, Miller GE. Psychological stress and disease. *JAMA.* 2007 Oct 10;298(14):1685–7.

Dusek JA, Otu HH, Wohlhueter AL, et al. Genomic counter-stress changes induced by the relaxation response. *PLoS One.* 2008 Jul 2;3(7):e2576.

Epel ES, Blackburn EH, Lin J, et al. Accelerated telomere shortening in response to life stress. Proc Natl Acad Sci U S A. 2004 Dec 7;101(49):17312-5. Epub 2004 Dec 1.

Funk RH, Monsees T, Ozkucur N. Electromagnetic effects: From cell biology to medicine. *Prog Histochem Cytochem.* 2009;43(4):177–264. Epub 2008 Sep 18.

Fitzpatrick AL, Standish LJ, Berger J, et al. Survival in HIV-1-positive adults practicing psychological or spiritual activities for one year. *Altern Ther Health Med.* 2007 Sep-Oct;13(5):18–20, 22–4.

Giltay EJ, Kamphuis MH, Kalmijn S, et al. Dispositional optimism and the risk of cardiovascular death: the Zutphen Elderly Study. *Arch Intern Med.* 2006 Feb 27;166(4):431–6.

Gordon JS, Staples JK, Blyta A, et al. Treatment of posttraumatic stress disorder in postwar Kosovar adolescents using mind-body skills groups: a randomized controlled trial. *J Clin Psychiatry.* 2008 Sep;69(9):1469–76.

Matthews KA, Räikkönen K, Sutton-Tyrrell K, Kuller LH. Optimistic attitudes protect against progression of carotid atherosclerosis in healthy middle-aged women. *Psychosom Med.* 2004 Sep-Oct;66(5):640–4.

Moritz S, Quan H, Rickhi B, et al. A home study-based spirituality education program decreases emotional distress and increases quality of life—a randomized, controlled trial. *Altern Ther Health Med.* 2006 Nov-Dec;12(6):26–35.

O'Donovan A, Lin J, Dhabhar FS, et al. Pessimism correlates with leukocyte telomere shortness and elevated interleukin-6 in postmenopausal women. *Brain Behav Immun.* 2009 May;23(4):446–9.

Rosenzweig S, Reibel DK, Greeson JM, et al. Mindfulness-based stress reduction is associated with improved glycemic control in type 2 diabetes mellitus: a pilot study. *Altern Ther Health Med.* 2007 Sep-Oct;13(5):36–8.

Torres SJ, Nowson CA. Relationship between stress, eating behavior, and obesity. *Nutrition.* 2007 Nov-Dec;23(11–12):887–94.

Chapter 3: The Tools of Quantum Healing

Anderson JW, Liu C, Kryscio RJ. Blood pressure response to transcendental meditation: a meta-analysis. *Am J Hypertens.* 2008 Mar;21(3):310–6.

Andrea H, Beurskens AJHM, Kant IJ, Davey GCL, Field AP, van Schayck CP. The relation between pathological worrying and fatigue in a working population. *J Psychosom Res.* 2004;57:399–407.

Bilkis MR, Mark KA. Mind-body medicine: practical applications in dermatology. *Arch Dermatol.* 1998;134:1437–1441.

Borkovec TD, Lyonfields JD, Wiser SL, Deihl L. The role of worrisome thinking in the suppression of cardiovascular response to phobic imagery. *Behav Res Ther.* 1993;31:321–324.

Brosschot JF, Thayer JF. Heart rate response is longer after negative emotions than after positive emotions. *Int J Psychophysiol.* 2003;50:181–187.

Burns JW, Holly A, Quartana P, et al. Trait anger management style moderates effects of actual ("state") anger regulation on symptom-specific reactivity and recovery among chronic low back pain patients. *Psychosom Med.* 2008 Oct;70(8):898-905.

Carrico DJ, Peters KM, Diokno AC. Guided imagery for women with interstitial cystitis: results of a prospective, randomized controlled pilot study. *J Altern Complement Med.* 2008 Jan-Feb;14(1):53–60.

DiPietro JA, Costigan KA, Nelson P, et al. Fetal responses to induced maternal relaxation during pregnancy. *Biol Psychol.* 2008 Jan;77(1):11–9. Epub 2007 Aug 31.

Goodhart DE. Some psychological effects associated with positive and negative thinking about stressful event outcomes: was Pollyanna right? *J Pers Soc Psychol.* 1985 Jan;48(1):216–32.

Graham JE, Lobel M, Glass P, Lokshina I. Effects of written anger expression in chronic pain patients: making meaning from pain. *J Behav Med.* 2008 Jun;31(3):201–12.

Howard J. Do Bach flower remedies have a role to play in pain control? A critical analysis investigating therapeutic value beyond the placebo effect, and the potential of Bach flower remedies as a psychological method of pain relief. *Complement Ther Clin Pract.* 2007 Aug;13(3):174–83.

Hu S, Bostow TR, Lipman DA, et al. Positive thinking reduces heart rate and fear responses to speech-phobic imagery. *Percept Mot Skills.* 1992 Dec;75(3 Pt 2):1067–73.

Hutcherson CA, Seppala EM, Gross JJ. Loving-kindness meditation increases social connectedness. *Emotion.* 2008 Oct;8(5):720–4.

Ishii H, Nagashima M, Tanno M, et al. Does being easily moved to tears as a response to psychological stress reflect response to treatment and the general prognosis in patients with rheumatoid arthritis? *Clin Exp Rheumatol.* 2003 Sep–Oct;21(5):61–6.

Jallo N, Bourguignon C, Taylor AG, et al. Stress management during pregnancy: designing and evaluating a mind-body intervention. *Fam Community Health.* 2008 Jul-Sep;31(3):190–203.

Kinnier RT, Hofsess C, Pongratz R, Lambert C. Attributions and affirmations for overcoming anxiety and depression. *Psychol Psychother.* 2009 Jun;82(Pt 2):153–69.

Lengacher CA, Bennett MP, Gonzalez L, et al. Immune responses to guided imagery during breast cancer treatment. *Biol Res Nurs.* 2008 Jan;9(3):205–14.

Linney BJ. Changing what goes on in your head: how to stop "ain't it awful?" *Physician Exec.* 2001 May–Jun;27(3):68–71.

Lipovetzky N, Hod H, Roth A, et al. Emotional events and anger at the workplace as triggers for a first event of the acute coronary syndrome: a case-crossover study. *Isr Med Assoc J.* 2007 Apr;9(4):310–5.

Lyonfields JD, Borkovec TD, Thayer JF. Vagal tone in generalized anxiety disorder and the effects of aversive imagery and worrisome thinking. Behav Ther. 1995;26:457–466.

McLaughlin KA, Borkovec TD, Sibrava NJ. The effects of worry and rumination on affect states and cognitive activity. *Behav Ther.* 2007 Mar;38(1):23–38. Epub 2006 Sep 25.

Menzies V, Kim S. Relaxation and guided imagery in Hispanic persons diagnosed with fibromyalgia: a pilot study. *Fam Community Health.* 2008 Jul–Sep;31(3):204–12.

Morone NE, Lynch CS, Greco CM, et al. "I felt like a new person." the effects of mindfulness meditation on older adults with chronic pain: qualitative narrative analysis of diary entries. *J Pain.* 2008 Sep;9(9):841-8.

Nunes DF, Rodriguez AL, da Silva Hoffmann F, et al. Relaxation and guided imagery program in patients with breast cancer undergoing radiotherapy is not associated with neuroimmunomodulatory effects. *J Psychosom Res.* 2007 Dec;63(6):647–55.

Pace TW, Negi LT, Adame DD, et al. Effect of compassion meditation on neuroendocrine, innate immune and behavioral responses to psychosocial stress. *Psychoneuroendocrinology.* 2009 Jan;34(1):87–98.

Peden AR, Rayens MK, Hall LA, Grant E. Testing an intervention to reduce negative thinking, depressive symptoms, and chronic stressors in low-income single mothers. *J Nurs Scholarsh.* 2005;37(3):268–74.

Philpot VD, Bamburg JW. Rehearsal of positive self-statements and restructured negative self-statements to increase self-esteem and decrease depression. *Psychol Rep.* 1996 Aug;79(1):83–91.

Pintov S, Hochman M, Livne A, et al. Bach flower remedies used for attention deficit hyperactivity disorder in children—a prospective double blind controlled study. *Eur J Paediatr Neurol.* 2005;9(6):395–8.

Schlotz W, Hellhammer J, Schulz P, Stone AA. Perceived work overload and chronic worrying predict weekend-weekday differences in the cortisol awakening response. *Psychosom Med.* 2004 Mar-Apr;66(2):207–14.

Segerstrom SC, Solomon GF, Kemeny ME, Fahey JL. Relationship of worry to immune sequelae of the Northridge earthquake. *J Behav Med.* 1998 Oct;21(5):433–50.

Shibeshi WA, Young-Xu Y, Blatt CM. Anxiety worsens prognosis in patients with coronary artery disease. *J Am Coll Cardiol.* 2007 May 22;49(20):2021-7. Epub 2007 May 4.

Stanton AL, Danoff-Burg S, Sworowski LA, et al. Randomized, controlled trial of written emotional expression and benefit finding in breast cancer patients. *J Clin Oncol.* 2002 Oct 15;20(20):4160-8.

Thomsen DK, Mehlsen MY, Christensen S, Zachariae R. Rumination: relationship with negative mood and sleep quality. *Pers Ind Dif.* 2003;34:1293–1301.

Thomsen DK, Mehlsen MY, Hokland M, Viidik A, Olesen F, Avlund K, et al. Negative thoughts and health: associations among rumination, immunity, and health care utilization in a young and elderly sample. *Psychosom Med.* 2004;66:363–371.

Trakhtenberg EC. The effects of guided imagery on the immune system: a critical review. *Int J Neurosci.* 2008 Jun;118(6):839–55.

Verplanken B, Friborg O, Wang CE, et al. Mental habits: metacognitive reflection on negative self-thinking. *J Pers Soc Psychol.* 2007 Mar;92(3):526–41.

Verplanken B, Velsvik R. Habitual negative body image thinking as psychological risk factor in adolescents. *Body Image.* 2008 Jun;5(2):133-40. Epub 2008 Jan 9.

Watanabe E, Fukuda S, Shirakawa T. Effects among healthy subjects of the duration of regularly practicing a guided imagery program. *BMC Complement Altern Med.* 2005 Dec 20;5:21.

Weigensberg MJ, Lane CJ, Winners O, et al. Acute effects of stress-reduction Interactive Guided Imagery(SM) on salivary cortisol in overweight Latino adolescents. *J Altern Complement Med.* 2009 Mar;15(3):297–303.

Watkins ER, Moulds M. Revealing negative thinking in recovered major depression: a preliminary investigation. *Behav Res Ther.* 2007 Dec;45(12):3069-76. Epub 2007 May 10.

Watkins ER. Constructive and unconstructive repetitive thought. *Psychol Bull.* 2008 Mar;134(2):163–206.

Weydert JA, Shapiro DE, Acra SA, et al. Evaluation of guided imagery as treatment for recurrent abdominal pain in children: a randomized controlled trial. *BMC Pediatr.* 2006 Nov 8;6:29.

Whiteside U, Chen E, Neighbors C, et al. Difficulties regulating emotions: Do binge eaters have fewer strategies to modulate and tolerate negative affect? *Eat Behav.* 2007 Apr;8(2):162–9.

Wilson RS, Krueger KR, Arnold SE, et al. Loneliness and risk of Alzheimer disease. *Arch Gen Psychiatry.* 2007 Feb;64(2):234–40.

Wynd CA. Guided health imagery for smoking cessation and long-term abstinence. *J Nurs Scholarsh.* 2005;37(3):245–50.

Part II: Your A to Z Guide to Healing Common Ailments

These references were used for determining the therapies listed in Part II.

Balch J. and Balch P. *Prescription for Nutritional Healing.* Garden City Park, NY: Avery Publishing Group, 1990.

Institute of Functional Medicine. *Textbook of Functional Medicine.* Boulder, CO: Johnson Printing, 2005.

Kaminski P. *Choosing Flower Essences: An Assessment Guide.* Nevada City, CA: Flower Essence Society, 1996.

Minich D. *Chakra Foods for Optimum Health: A Guide to the Foods that can Improve Your Energy, Inspire Creative Changes, Open Your Heart, and Heal Body, Mind, and Spirit.* San Francisco: Conari Press, 2009.

Minich D. *Quantum Supplements: A Total Health and Wellness Makeover with Vitamins, Minerals, and Herbs.* San Francisco: Conari Press, 2009.

Murray M. and Pizzorno J. *Encyclopedia of Natural Medicine.* 2nd ed. Rocklin, CA: Prima Publishing, 1998.

Pizzorno L., Pizzorno J., and Murray M. *Natural Medicine Instructions for Patients.* London: Elsevier Science, 2002.

Resources

Recommended Books

Chakras

Dale C. *The Subtle Body: An Encyclopedia of Your Energetic Anatomy.* Boulder, CO: Sounds True, 2009.

Dale C. *New Chakra Healing: the Revolutionary 32-Center Energy System.* St. Paul, MN: Llewellyn Publications, 1998.

Myss C. *Anatomy of the Spirit: The Seven Stages of Power and Healing.* London: Bantam Books, 1996.

Rippentrop B. and Adamson E. *The Complete Idiot's Guide to Chakras.* New York, NY: Penguin Group, 2009.

Emotions

Hawkins D. *Power vs. Force: The Hidden Determinants of Human Behavior.* Sedona, AZ: Veritas Publishing, 2004.

Empowered Living: Affirmations

Hay L. *I Love My Body.* Santa Monica, CA: Hay House, Inc. 1985.

Hay L. *You Can Heal Your Life.* Carlsbad, CA: Hay House, Inc., 1984.

Levine B. *Your Body Believes Every Word You Say: The Language of the Body/Mind Connection.* Fairfield, CT: Words Work Press, 2000.

Shapiro D. *Your Body Speaks Your Mind: Decoding the Emotional, Psychological, and Spiritual Messages That Underlie Illness.* Boulder, CO: Sounds True, 2006.

Flower Essences

Gurudas. *Flower Essences and Vibrational Healing.* San Rafael, CA: Cassandra Press, 1989.

Kaminski P. *Choosing Flower Essences: An Assessment Guide.* Nevada City, CA: Flower Essence Society, 1996.

Stein D. *Healing with Flower and Gemstone Essences.* Freedom, CA: The Crossing Press, 1996.

Health and Healing

Myss C. and Shealy CN. *The Creation of Health: The Emotional, Psychological, and Spiritual Responses That Promote Health and Healing.* New York: Three Rivers Press, 1988.

Soames P. *The Essence of Self-Healing: How to Bring Health and Happiness Into Your Life.* Spring, TX: FleetStreet Publications, 2000.

Shamanic Practices and Philosophy

Andrews T. *Animal-Wise: The Spirit Language and Signs of Nature.* Jackson, TN: Dragonhawk Publishing, 1999.

Arrien A. *The Four-Fold Way: Walking the Paths of the Warrior, Teacher, Healer and Visionary.* San Francisco: Harper San Francisco, 1993.

Harner M. *The Way of the Shaman.* New York: Bantam Books, 1980.

Visualization

Gawain S. *Creative Visualization: Use the Power of Your Imagination to Create What You Want in Your Life.* Novato, CA: Nataraj Publishing, 2002.

Websites

Bach Flower Remedies, *www.bachflower.com*, 1-800-214-2850.
Flower Essences Services, *www.fesflowers.com*, 1-800-548-0075.

Index

Abandonment, 155
Acetyl-L-carnitine, 159, 197
Acknowledgment, desire for, 97
Acne, 45–46
Addictions, 46–48
Adrenal fatigue, 49–51
Aggression, 176, 219
Aging, 51–52
Agrimony, 168, 170, 214
Alcoholism, 53–55
Allergies, 55–57
Aloe Vera, 59, 77, 115, 123
Aloe Vera juice, 96
Aloneness, 55. See also Loneliness
Alopecia areata (hair loss), 132–134
Alpha lipoic acid, 178, 197
Alpine Lily, 83, 177, 184, 210
Anemia, 15, 57–58
Angelica, 108, 127, 178, 189, 206
Angel's Trumpet, 63, 96, 142, 172, 233
Anger, 45, 59–60, 65, 70, 77, 83, 90,
    97, 99, 103, 115, 117, 130, 135, 138,
    140, 142, 161, 170, 172, 178, 187,
    199, 213, 216, 231, 233, 236. See
    also Rage
Antioxidants, 246
Anxiety, 60–63, 124, 126, 128, 132, 151,
    182, 250
Apathy, 57, 79, 136, 250
Appetite, excessive, 108–110

Apple cider vinegar, 157
Apple pectin. See Pectin
Apprehension, 165
Arginine, 138
Arnica, 81, 174
Arthritis
    osteoarthritis, 198–200
    rheumatoid arthritis, 216–218
Artichoke, 121
Ashwagandha, 49
Aspects of being, 14
Aspen, 61, 68, 128, 165, 187, 207
Asthma, 63–65
Astragalus, 49
Atherosclerosis, 65–67
Atopic dermatitis, 104–106
Attention-deficit (hyperactivity)
    disorder (ADD, ADHD), 67–69
Autoimmune conditions, 15–16
Autoimmune disease, 70–72

Baby Blue Eyes, 72, 127, 201
Bach, Edward, 30
Back pain, 72–74
Baldness, 132–134
Barberry, 250
Basil, 210, 242
B-complex vitamin. See Vitamin B
    complex
Beech, 85, 94, 214

Bee-pollen granules, 55
Benign prostatic hyperplasia, 211–213
Beta-carotene, 63, 130
Betaine HCI, 157
Betaine hydrochloric acid, 75, 213, 216
Beta-sitosterol, 211
Bifidobacterium bifidum, 165
Bilberry, 149, 240
Bilkis, Michael R., 26
Binge eating, 23, 85–86. *See also* Eating
   disorders/problems
Bioflavonoids, 55, 63, 72, 81, 94, 142,
   144, 161, 174, 182, 187, 199, 223,
   231, 236, 239
Biotin, 132, 197, 226
Bitter melon, 149
Bitterness, 172, 199
Black Cohosh, 101, 140, 182, 209
Blackberry, 66, 96, 111, 142, 147, 174,
   178, 240
Black-eyed Susan, 87, 98, 172
Bladder infection, 235–237
Bleeding Heart, 124, 138
Blindness, 246–247
Bloating (abdominal), 74–76
Blood pressure, 8, 9, 41
   high, 27, 76–79
   low, 79–80
Blood sugar, high (hyperglycemia),
   149–151
Body, web interconnecting, 4–5
Body function, 39
Body-mind therapies, 6, 8–9
Body-mind-spirit revolution, 6–9, 7
Bone healing (fracture or break),
   80–82
Borage, 138
Boswellia, 119, 161, 174, 199, 221
Breast cancer, 22, 38, 39
Breast problems, 82–85
Brittleness, 97
Bromelain, 55, 63, 122, 199, 216, 221,
   223
Bulimia, 85–86. *See also* Eating
   disorders/problems
Bunions, 119–120
Burdock, 45
Burning up, emotion of, 140

Butterbur, 134, 187
Buttercup, 79, 206, 229

Calcium, 61, 77, 81, 119, 140, 151, 163,
   184, 190, 195, 200–201, 209, 221
Calendula, 138, 153, 177
California Pitcher Plant, 108, 127, 197
California Poppy, 92, 119, 221
California Wild Rose, 90, 108, 153
Callousness, 65
Cancer, 87–90. *See also* Breast cancer
Candida Albicans overgrowth,
   249–252
Cardiovascular disease, 21
Carpal tunnel syndrome, 90–91
Cayenne, 79
Celiac disease, 91–93
Centaury, 94, 117
Cerato, 92, 106, 180
Chakras, 11–18, *13, 14*
Chamomile, 98, 140, 165, 184, 189, 248
Chaparral, 106, 124
Chasteberry, 159, 182, 209
Cherry Plum, 49, 77, 132, 149, 163, 187,
   191, 225
Chestnut Bud, 182
Chicory, 85
Chlamydia (venereal disease), 241–244
Cholesterol, high, 146–149
Choline, 233
Chondroitin, 174, 199
Chromium, 45, 149, 159, 203, 205
Chrysanthemum, 168
Cinnamon, 149, 159, 203, 231
Clematis, 94, 117, 147, 149, 151
Coenzyme Q10, 77, 130, 134, 159, 231
Cold, common, 93–95
Coldness, 197
Common cold, 93–95
Competition, 184
Conflict, 97
Constipation, 95–97
Copper, 153
Cordyceps, 49
Corn, 55, 119, 130, 144
Cortisol, 9, 27, 38, 49
Cosmos, 136, 170
Coughing, 97–99

Crab Apple, 189
Criticalness, 199
Crown chakra, 13, 17, 40–41
Curcumin, 119, 161, 174, 199, 216
Cysts, in breast, 82–85

Dandelion, 45, 66, 121, 149
Davis, Adelle, 5
Deerbrush, 231
Defeat, 153
Defensiveness, 55, 144
Deglycyrrhizinated licorice (DGL), 225
Denial, 68, 136, 180, 193, 213, 246
Depletion, 149
Depression, 21, 25, 28, 33–34, 59, 79,
    99–100, 128, 178
Despair, 51, 124, 178, 180, 211
Devil's claw, 72
Diabetes, 149–151
Diarrhea, 100–102
Digestive enzymes, 20, 70, 72, 75, 108,
    140, 157, 161, 174, 189, 199. See also
    pancreatic enzymes
Dill, 55, 68, 75, 92, 105, 140, 157, 165,
    227
Disappointment, 240
Discomfort, 157
Disconnection, 99, 119
Disease, path to, 5
Distance, 197
Distant, being, 124
Distraction, 119
Distrust, 126
Docosahexaenoic acid (DHA), 197, 207
Dogwood, 77, 101, 117, 121, 172, 174,
    191, 199, 201, 225
Dong quai, 182, 209
Doubt, 68, 203, 211, 221
Doubt, self-, 165
Dread, 61, 246, 248

Ear infection, 102–104
Easter Lily, 184, 210
Eating disorders/problems, 85–86,
    106–108, 108–110
Echinacea, 81, 87, 98, 191
Echinacea purpurea root, 94

Eczema, 104–106
Eicosapentaenoic acid, 197
Electrolytes, 3
Elm, 72, 142, 191, 195, 227
Emotion identification, 21–26
Emotional attachment, 238
Emotional eating, 106–108. See also
    Eating disorders/problems
Emotional exhaustion, 101
Emotional extremes, 101
Emotional states, 23, 24
Emotions. See also individual emotions
    flower essences and, 32
    repressed, 25
    toxic, 233
    unexpressed, 106
Emptiness, 101
Energy system, 11, 12
Enlarged prostate, 211–213
Enzymes, pancreatic, 92, 213, 216, 238.
    See also Digestive enzymes
Esophageal reflux, 140–142
Estrogen, 82
Eucalyptus, 231
Evening Primrose, 70, 138, 149, 159,
    177
Excessive appetite, 108–110
Exhaustion. See Fatigue
Eyesight
    farsightedness, 110–112
    nearsightedness, 193–195
    vision loss, 246–247

Fairy Lantern, 68, 195
Farsightedness, 110–112
Fatigue, 25, 28, 112–114
Fatty acids. See Omega-3 fatty acids
Fatty liver (liver problems), 178–180
Fear, 23, 49, 61, 63, 87, 96, 106, 111,
    113, 117, 132, 135, 140, 142, 151,
    155, 174, 182, 189, 190, 194, 195,
    197, 203, 206, 207, 211, 221, 226,
    229, 248
Feelings, accumulation of, 147
Fenugreek, 149
Fever, 115–116
Feverfew, 134, 187

Fiber supplements, 83, 96, 101, 120, 142, 146, 149, 157, 205, 233, 238, 239–240, 250
Fibromyalgia, 38, 116–118
Fight-or-flight feeling, 151
Filaree, 75, 128, 165, 194, 248
Fish oil, 45, 53, 70, 72, 92, 99, 104, 119, 122, 124, 138, 142, 159, 180, 184, 189, 205, 209, 211, 213, 238, 246
5-hydroxytryptophan (5-HTP), 99, 117, 135, 163
Flaxseed meal, ground, 83
Flaxseed oil, 45, 53, 70, 72, 92, 99, 104, 119, 122, 124, 142, 159, 180, 184, 189, 209, 211, 213, 238, 246
Flower essences, 16, 30–32. See also *individual flower essences*
Flu (viral infection), 244–246
Folate, 57, 79
Folic acid, 51, 57, 65, 122, 130, 136, 172
Foot pain, 119–120
Forget-me-not, 189
Fragility, feeling of, 201
Fright, 207. *See also* Fear
Frustration, 59, 77, 130, 170, 209, 211
Fuchsia, 106, 177
Fulfillment, lack of, 85, 106
Fury, 59, 121, 142

Gallstones, 120–122
Gamma linolenic acid, 197
Garlic, 65, 77, 146, 207, 231, 244, 250
Genes, 9
Genital warts (venereal disease), 241–244
Gentian, 47
Ginger, 70, 72, 119, 134, 161, 174, 187, 199, 216, 221, 231
Ginger root extract, 192
Ginkgo, 149
Ginkgo biloba, 63, 180
Glucosamine, 174, 199
Glucosamine sulfate, 170
Golden Ear Drops, 121, 161
Goldenrod, 70, 206, 216
Goldenseal, 213, 231, 236, 250
Gonorrhea (venereal disease), 241–244
Gorse, 127, 201, 248

Gout, 122–124
Grape seed, 240
Grape seed extract, 65, 149
Green tea extract, 104, 159, 167, 203
Grief, 97, 108, 117, 124–126, 138, 223
Grounding (feeling ungrounded or detached from life), 126–128
Guar gum, 83, 96, 101, 120, 142, 146
Guided imagery. *See* Visualizations
Guilt, 106, 128–129, 209, 242
Gum disease, 129–132
Gymnema, 149

Hair loss, 132–134
Hammertoes, 119–120
Hawthorn, 61
Headaches, 134–136, 186–188
Health, path to, *5*
Hearing loss, 136–138
Heart chakra, 13, 16, 30–32
Heart disease, 15, 138–140
Heartburn, 140–142
Heather, 128, 130, 155
Helplessness, 51, 90, 121, 155
Hemorrhoids, 142–144
Hepatitis (liver problems), 178–180
Herpes simplex virus (viral infection, venereal disease), 241–244, 244–246
Hesperidin, 142, 182
Hibiscus, 210, 242
High blood cholesterol, 146–149
High blood pressure, 27, 76–79. *See also* Blood pressure
High blood sugar (hyperglycemia), 149–151
Hives (urticaria), 144–146
Holly, 138, 184, 219
Honeysuckle, 47, 66, 142, 161, 172, 193
Hopelessness, 53, 178
Hops, 61, 163, 248
Hops extract, 70
Hornbeam, 94, 149, 182, 233
Horse chestnut, 240
Human Immunodeficiency Virus (viral infection), 244–246
Huperzine A, 180

Hurt (emotion of), 83, 85, 87, 138, 223, 238, 244
Hydrochloric acid, 157
Hyperactivity, 67–69
Hypercholesterolemia (high blood cholesterol), 146–149
Hyperglycemia, 149–151
Hypertension, 76–79, 149
Hyperthyroidism, 151–153
Hypotension, 79–80
Hypothyroidism, 153–155

Immune system, 17. *See also* Autoimmune disease
Impatiens, 123
Impotence (infertility), 159–160
Inability to move forward, 123
Inability to "take it all in," 92
Inadequacy, 47, 83, 126, 149, 159, 189, 206
Inauthenticity, feeling of, 103
Incontinence, urinary, 155–156
Indecision, 121
Indian Paintbrush, 90, 159, 177, 203, 212
Indian Pink, 75, 157, 180, 197
Indigestion, 156–158
Infertility, 159–160
Inflammation, 161–162
Inflammation, emotion of, 123, 142, 231
Inflexibility, 65
Infuriation, feeling of, 123
Inositol, 203
Insecurity, 47, 81, 92, 119, 123, 126, 130, 142, 144, 155, 159, 176, 182, 189, 206, 219, 244
Insomnia, 162–165
Integrity, loss of, 155
Interconnecting web within body, 4–5, 4
Interstitial cystitis (IC, urinary tract infection), 38, 235–237
Intimacy, fear of, 138
Invasion, feeling of, 94, 236
Iris, 90, 135, 159
Iron, 57, 132, 153, 184, 238
Irritability, 25

Irritable bowel syndrome (IBS), 165–167
Irritation, 59, 90, 104, 115, 136, 161, 165, 167, 187, 209, 211, 236
Isolation, 47, 51, 53, 55, 68
Itching, 167–169

Jaundice (liver problems), 178–180
Jaw tightness (temporomandibular joint, TMJ), 170–171
Jealousy, 184

Kidney stones, 172–174
Knee pain, 174–176

Lactobacillus acidophilus, 165
Lactobacillus GG, 101
Lactobacillus thamnosus, 101
Lady's Slipper, 149, 195
Larch, 121, 144, 199, 206, 229
Larkspur, 119, 153, 219
Lavender, 132, 135, 163, 187
L-carnitine, 151, 159
Lecithin (phosphatidylcholine), 120
Left-side-of-body complaints, 176–178
Licorice, 104, 178, 182, 209, 225
Licorice root, 49, 63
Limiting beliefs, 26–29, 34
Liver problems, 178–180
Loneliness, 99, 108, 124. *See also* Aloneness
Longing, 108
Lotus, 178
Love, 23
Low blood pressure, 79–80. *See also* Blood pressure
Lumps, in breast, 82–85
Lutein, 246
Lysine supplements, 242

Madia, 68
Magnesium, 61, 63, 65, 77, 81, 96, 117, 119, 134, 136, 138, 140, 163, 172, 184, 187, 190, 195, 207, 209, 221, 247
Mallow, 178, 189
Manzanita, 47
Mariposa Lily, 83, 177, 182

Mark, Kenneth A., 26
Meditations, crown chakra and, 40–41
Melatonin, 163
Memory loss, 180–181
Menopause, 182–184
Menstrual difficulties, 184–186
Migraines, 186–188. *See also*
  Headaches
Milk thistle, 53, 121, 178
Milk thistle extract, 238
Mimulus, 135, 138, 149, 163
Mind-dump exercise, 28–29
Mindful eating, 17, 47
Mineral supplement, 126
Moods, changing, 209
Morning Glory, 101, 113, 151, 182, 184
Morning sickness, 192–193
Motion sickness, 192–193
Mountain Pride, 57, 157, 206, 219
Mugwort, 117, 197
Multiple sclerosis, 188–190
Muscle tightness, 190–192
Mustard, 99, 124, 223
Myopia, 193–195

N-acetylcysteine, 178
Nasturtium, 135
Nausea, 192–193
Nearsightedness (myopia), 193–195
Neck pain, 195–196
Neem, 45, 231
Negative thought repetition, 26–29
Nervousness, 189
Neurotransmitters, 3–4
Niacin, 51, 65, 138, 146
Notice, desire for, 97
Nourishment, root chakra and, 19–21
Numbness, 197–198
Numbness, emotion of, 124

Oak, 72, 94, 113
Oat bran, 96, 101, 142
Obesity, 205–207
Olive, 57
Omega-3 fatty acids, 21, 45, 53, 63, 70,
  72, 92, 99, 104, 119, 122, 124, 138,
  142, 159, 180, 184, 189, 213, 216
Oregon Grape, 30, 197, 201, 207, 250

Osteoarthritis, 198–200
Osteoporosis, 200–203
Otitis media, 102–104
Ovarian cysts, 203–205
Overweight (obesity), 205–207
Overwhelmed, feeling of being, 72, 75,
  77, 85, 92, 94, 115, 132, 147, 149,
  163, 165, 167, 180, 250

Pain
  emotional, 161
  visualizations and, 38–39
Pancreatic enzymes, 92, 213, 216, 238
Panic attacks, 207–209
Pantothenic acid, 170
Papain, 55, 221
Passionflower, 61, 163, 248
Pectin, 83, 96, 101, 120, 142, 146, 233
Penstemon, 111, 180
Peppermint, 113, 117, 135, 187
Peppermint oil, 165
Periodontal Disease, 129–132
Periodontitis, 129–132
Phosphatidylcholine (lecithin), 120
Phosphatidylserine, 180
Pine, 128, 199
Pine bark extract, 65, 240
Pink Monkeyflower, 144
Pink Yarrow, 83, 250
Polycystic Ovarian Syndrome, 203–205
Pomegranate, 210
Potassium, 190, 195
Power animals, 29–30
Premenstrual syndrome (PMS),
  209–211
Preoccupation, 163
Pretty Face, 45, 206
Primrose oil, 45
Probiotics, 70, 75, 92, 101, 130, 157,
  165, 167, 205, 216, 236, 242, 250
Prostate problems, 211–213
Prostatitis, 211–213
Protein supplements, 126, 151
Proteins, role of, 5
Psoriasis, 213–215
Psyllium, 83, 96, 101, 120, 142, 146,
  233, 239, 250
Pumpkin seed oil, 211

Quantum healing, description of, 3
Quantum healing wheel, 15–18
Queen Anne's Lace, 111, 194, 246
Quercetin, 55, 63, 104, 119, 122, 144, 174, 182, 199, 216, 221, 223, 231
Quince, 72, 117

Rabbitbrush, 51, 140, 193
Rage, 59, 99, 121, 123, 140, 161, 170. *See also* Anger
Red Chestnut, 238, 250
Red Clover, 170
Refusal, 193
Regret, 85, 128, 244
Rejection, 153, 159, 197
Reluctance, 174
Repression, 236
Resentment, 199, 201, 216
Rheumatoid arthritis, 22, 216–218
Rhodiola rosea, 49
Right-side-of-body complaints, 218–221
Rigidity, 172
Root chakra, 13, 15, 19–21
Rosemary, 68, 127, 168

Sacral chakra, 13, 15, 21–26
Sadness, 124, 209, 238
Sage, 123
Sagebrush, 142, 165
Saguaro, 130, 212
Saw palmetto, 211
Scarlet Monkeyflower, 103, 161, 170, 178
Sciatica, 221–222
Scleranthus, 130, 201, 214
Scotch Broom, 53, 124
Selenium, 70, 153, 178
Self-containment, 87
Self-doubt, 165
Self-suppression, 87
Separation, 138
Serotonin, 3–5
Sexually transmitted disease (venereal disease), 241–244
Shame, 45, 106, 113, 128, 213, 229, 242
Shasta Daisy, 140, 194
Shyness, 144

Siberian ginseng, 49
Silence, uncomfortable, 25
Silica, 132
Silymarin, 167, 178, 213
Sinus congestion, 222–224
Skin irritation
    hives, 144–146
    itching, 167–169
    psoriasis, 213–215
Snapdragon, 170
Solar plexus chakra, 13, 15–16, 26–29, 29–30
Soreness, in breast, 82–85
St. John's Wort, 99, 184
Stagnation, 142, 147, 199
Star of Bethlehem, 121, 135, 191
Star Tulip, 103, 136, 197
Sticky Monkeyflower, 159, 210, 242
Stiffness, emotional, 65
Stifled, feeling of being, 195
Stomach pain, 25
Stomach problems
    heartburn, 140–142
    indigestion, 156–158
    stomach ulcers, 224–226
Stress, 28, 33, 38, 226–229
Strife, 172
Stuck, feeling of being, 174
Stuttering, 229–230
Sunflower, 149, 210
Supplements, 19–21. See also *individual supplements*
Support, lack of, 72, 81, 155
Sweet Chestnut, 51, 99
Sweet Pea, 81, 92
Syphilis (venereal disease), 241–244

Tansy, 203
Temporomandibular joint, 170–171
Tension, 187, 190, 209
Third eye chakra, 13, 17, 35–40
Thoughts, impact of, 27
Threatened, feeling of being, 126
Throat chakra, 13, 16–17, 32–35
Thyroid. *See* Hyperthyroidism; Hypothyroidism
Tiger Lily, 203, 210, 212
Tight throat, 25

TMJ, 170–171
Tooth pain, 231–232
Toxin overload, 232–235
Transcendental meditation, 41
Trillium, 123
Trumpet Vine, 103, 229
Trust, lack of, 72, 96
Turbulence, 101
Turmeric, 70, 72, 121, 161, 178, 231

Ulcers, 140–142, 224–226
Uncertainty, 151
Uneasiness, 157, 193
Untrusting, feeling of being, 72, 96
Unworthiness, 113
Urinary tract infection, 235–237
Urticaria, 144–146
Uterine fibroids, 237–239
Uva ursi, 236

Valerian, 61, 163, 248
Varicose veins, 239–241
Venereal disease (sexually transmitted disease), 241–244
Vinegar, apple cider, 157
Viral infection, 244–246
Vision loss, 246–247. See also Eyesight
Visualizations, third eye chakra and, 35–40
Vitamin A, 45, 103, 104, 111, 130, 151, 153, 194, 213, 225, 236, 242, 244
Vitamin B complex, 45, 47, 49, 53, 61, 72, 77, 79, 92, 99, 104, 113, 132, 134, 138, 159, 163, 170, 172, 184, 187, 197, 207, 213, 221, 226, 233, 242, 247
Vitamin B1, 221
Vitamin B2, 153
Vitamin B3, 153
Vitamin B5, 170, 226

Vitamin B6, 153, 197, 221, 226
Vitamin B12, 51, 57, 79
Vitamin C, 45, 49, 55, 57, 61, 63, 65, 70, 72, 77, 81, 94, 96, 103, 104, 111, 113, 120, 130, 132, 138, 142, 144, 151, 153, 161, 170, 178, 182, 187, 194, 207, 213, 216, 223, 225, 226, 231, 233, 236, 239, 242, 244, 246
Vitamin D, 20, 45, 70, 104, 119, 189, 200, 213
Vitamin E, 45, 65, 77, 104, 111, 120, 130, 132, 138, 151, 159, 194, 213, 216, 246
Vitamin K, 81, 172, 201
Vulnerability, 92, 184, 189, 201

Walnut, 66, 96, 147, 172, 193, 223, 236
Web, interconnecting, 4–5, 4
Weighed down, feeling of being, 147
White Chestnut, 68, 99, 135, 163
White willow bark, 231
Wild Oat, 99
Willow, 77, 87, 123, 191, 193, 216
Willow bark, 72
Willow bark, white, 231
Withdrawal, 147
Worry, 61, 75, 128, 135, 163, 190, 209, 225, 247–249

Xylitol, 103

Yarrow, 16, 144, 151, 155, 250
Yeast infection, 249–252
Yerba Santa, 98, 223

Zinc, 20, 45, 70, 81, 94, 103, 104, 111, 130, 132, 153, 161, 194, 211, 213, 216, 225, 236, 242, 244, 246
Zinnia, 138, 149, 159

About the Author

Deanna M. Minich, PhD, CN, is a nutrition educator and researcher active in the healing arts for nearly twenty years. She is the author of three previous books: *Chakra Foods for Optimum Health, Quantum Supplements*, and *An A-Z Guide to Food Additives*, and holds a Master of Science degree in human nutrition from the University of Illinois at Chicago and a doctorate in medical sciences/human nutrition from the University of Groningen in The Netherlands. Deanna's integrated, unique approach to health and healing comes from 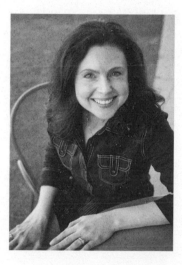 combining academic training with many years of study of energetic modalities such as shamanic healing, Reiki, and yoga. You can read more about Deanna and her work at *www.foodandspirit.com*.